menopause

Edited by MK Czerwiec

graphic mundi

menopause

a comic treatment

contents

acknowledgments

This is the first anthology I've edited, and it's been a learning experience. Editing an anthology is something that, in the idea stage, feels very straightforward, but in execution it isn't. Thank you to each of the artists in this volume for their willingness, timeliness, enthusiasm, patience, and encouragement.

Thank you to Susan Squier for advice, insight, editing, and role modeling; to Ann Fox for her great mind and generous spirit; to Kendra Boileau for believing in and supporting this project from my first mention of it; to Nicola Streeten for additional resources and encouragement (and for being Nicola); to Judith A. Houck for historical background on the treatment of women during perimenopause; to Peggy Mason for information on the neurology of menopause; to Mita Mahato and Sarah Leavitt for always having my back; to our amazing worldwide Graphic Medicine community who inspire me every day; and to my wife Cindy, once again, for everything.

introduction

MK Czerwiec

My mother died when she was ninety-three years old, in October of my forty-ninth year. Her older sister died in March of my fiftieth year. Caring for the two of them had consumed much of my time, and my identity, for the preceding decade. Once they were both gone, the way my life suddenly changed was disorienting. Because I had also helped care for my disabled father and had worked as a nurse, much of my life had revolved around caregiving responsibilities. But after the death of my mother and my aunt, and for the first time since I was seventeen years old, no person was looking to me for care. No one needed my help with checkbooks, groceries, dressing, errands, house maintenance, the bathroom. No more weekly anxious morning drives to the western suburbs of Chicago or exhausted, late-night drives home. No more desperate phone calls between visits requiring me to vacate my life to salvage theirs.

Then, in April of my fiftieth year, hot flashes arrived—and with them came weight gain, palpitations, sudden bouts of sadness, fatigue, bloating, unexplained agitation, swollen feet, food cravings, random anxiety, and tingling hands. Which was more disorienting, my elder-care empty nest or this cascade of symptoms that culminated with my bursting into a profuse sweat every fifteen minutes?

It didn't matter, because it was all happening at once. It became impossible to separate the symptoms of grieving from the symptoms of perimenopause, the emotional from the hormonal. I felt like I was being pulled into a dark abyss.

I also felt woefully unprepared for all of this.

Eventually, I did what I have done in previous challenging times of my life: I turned to popular culture. More specifically, I turned to comics. Unfortunately, the comics I could find about menopause were not very helpful, and sometimes they were even hurtful. Most of them were either single-panel jokes about hot flashes or expressions of this or that symptom of perimenopause as an inconvenience to a husband or a male partner. Instead of feeling seen and empowered, I felt further isolated and belittled.

The first (and only, as far as I can tell) book-length collection of comics about menopause seems to have appeared in 1950 and was titled *Minnie Pauses to Reflect*, by Nora Preddy. The dedication of Preddy's forty-panel collection of single-page comics sets the tone for the work. It reads, "To my husband for his patience with me in mine."

The women in *Minnie Pauses* are frequently portrayed as judging one another

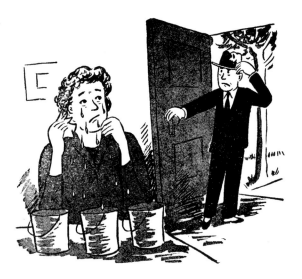

TILLIE THE TEARFUL

He: "Buckets of tears! Buckets of tears! Why don't you dry up? I've tried everything. Now I'm going home to Mother! Good-by!"

She: "Boo-hoo-hoo-hooooooo oo o!"

for inappropriate management of symptoms (not seeking surgery or taking hormone medications, eating or drinking excessively). Most of the comics demonstrate how inconvenient perimenopausal women are for just about everyone around them, particularly the men in their lives.

A new collection of comics was needed—one that shared stories that might actually be helpful, stories that encourage those of us facing the symptoms of perimenopause to find our voices rather than remain silent, to invite us into strength rather than push us further into shame. Thanks to the incredible energy of the growing Graphic Medicine community, the people who were perfectly suited to create this new collection of comics about menopause were a visit to social media, a website, or an email away.

I asked my comics idols and cherished colleagues to help me out. I asked powerful and inspiring role models who are going

through menopause, or who have already been through it, to make comics about their experiences and about how they coped. This book collects those responses. The comics in this collection represent a range of life experiences, professions, ages, gender and sexual identities, ethnicities, and health states.

I feel deep gratitude not only for the wonderful comics in this collection but also for what the contributors shared about what they gained from making these comics. For some, these are the first comics they have made. Others, who have been making comics for years reported that this one was different. Many expressed being changed by the process, as their understanding of menopause was deepened by the experience of drawing about it.

Managing this time of our lives takes a team. We feel as though we go through menopause alone, but that's only true if we allow it to be. Constantly struggling to pull ourselves out of torpor, stiffness, and ache is not easy work. We need to be supportive of one another and of ourselves. I was fortunate enough to find an older therapist, who has the vitality of a woman who has survived menopause, and a young athletic trainer, who has the advantage of not really knowing that any of it is coming. After I established a support system, more life change required that I move two states away. In doing this I realized the importance (and fragile nature) of my new support system. My period returned after a five-month hiatus, as did the fatigue, grief, food cravings, seeking comfort in drinking—all of it—and I felt alone. Again. I'm now remembering what helps and what doesn't, and finding the will to reach out. Again.

We need to help one another brainstorm effective strategies for coping with menopause, knowing that there will be many different paths, many ups and downs. The comics in this collection testify to the importance of sharing our stories. My hope is that the work that appears in this collection can begin to offer a community of support. While it may be comforting to find humor in the absurdity of some of our symptoms, it's important to remember that menopause itself isn't a joke. Comparing stories—and breaking the silence around menopause—in ways that make us feel safe, valued, and empowered is important. It's freeing, and feeling free makes challenging things easier, giving us the communal space in which to find our own styles for living through the challenges of perimenopause. I hope this book of comics will be conducive to finding and embracing one's own style, the way artists must do for their work.

My artistic and academic work has been informed and deepened by perspectives arising from the disability rights movement, particularly by the idea of *adaptation*, which asks: How do we adapt to the bodies we find ourselves in? How must our adaptations change with our bodies over time? Portrait artist and disability rights activist Riva Lehrer writes in her August 2017 *New York Times* op-ed piece, "Where All Bodies Are Exquisite," that "the magical thing about bodies [is that] they respond to the unexpected with their own forms of poetic genius." The symptoms of approaching menopause *feel* unexpected and unpredictable. Most of us aren't told about the complexities of what is coming. We are left searching for a trail of clues leading to an

understanding of our own bodies and what they are doing.

We can benefit greatly from teaching and learning truths about our bodies, such as how menopause works for a range of individuals and how we can find ways to adapt. What better medium than comics to do this important work? Comics have a long history of taking on stigmatized topics. They make literal the metaphors we use to describe our bodies, and they can be playful and enjoyable, even if the topic they tackle is not. Most of all, comics give us a sense of community. The work that Graphic Medicine does so well is crucial because it pulls the focus away from what one person (you, or I) needs to do to manage menopause. Rather than making it a problem of the individual (as in Preddy's comics), Graphic Medicine allows us to focus on understanding how the knowledge we gain as a collective, and the options this opens for us, can move us from isolation to community, from problem to poetic genius.

When my mother was descending into the dementia that dominated her last few years, her parting words to me were always, "Take care of yourself." Though I appreciated her thoughtfulness, I also wondered what message she was actually trying to send me. Was it some kind of warning arising from her life regrets? Her advice also frustrated me. I had heard the same words as a nurse—that to survive prioritizing the needs of others over our own needs, we should "take care of ourselves." But what does this really mean? Get manicures and occasional massages? Buy a fancy new pair of shoes now and then? Have a glass or three of wine every night? (There is constant messaging around us to self-soothe with alcohol. For an eye-opening examination of this phenomenon, see *Drink: The Intimate Relationship Between Women and Alcohol* by Ann Dowsett Johnston.) Too many of us are forced to resort to quick ways of numbing ourselves because that is the easiest thing to do, and we don't have the time or energy for more than what we are already doing.

How can we instead invite ourselves to respond to menopause with poetic genius? How can we respond with style? How can I adapt the way I have tried to generously love others in my life to how I love myself? How can I revise my life's role models away from women who perhaps felt their only option for survival was to give themselves away, or to judge their own and others' failures, toward people who know their worth, possess their own power, and support one another?

These comics are, I hope, a strong push in that direction. There are more to be made. Consider picking up a pen and trying one.

Now that's taking care of yourself.

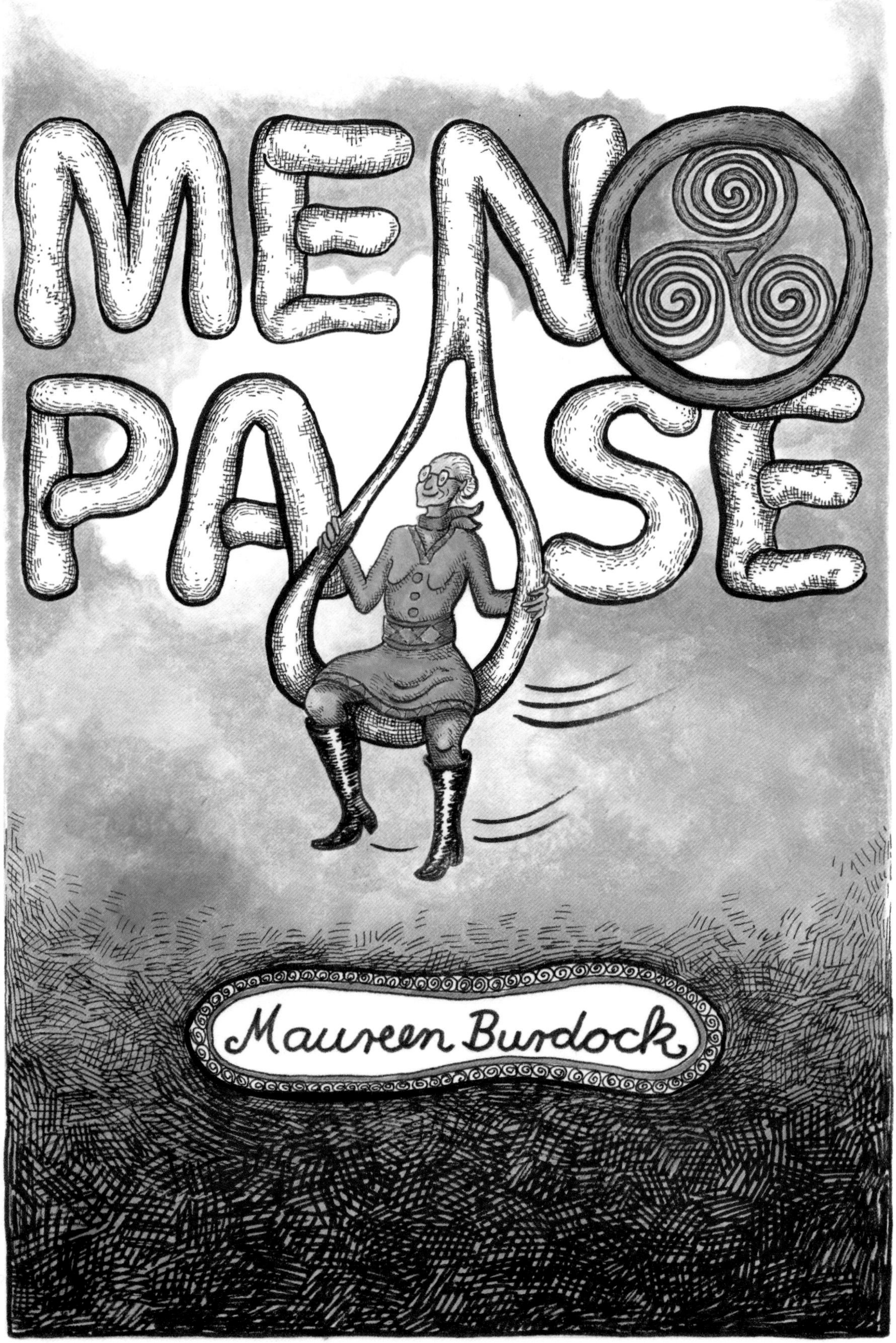
MENOPAUSE
Maureen Burdock

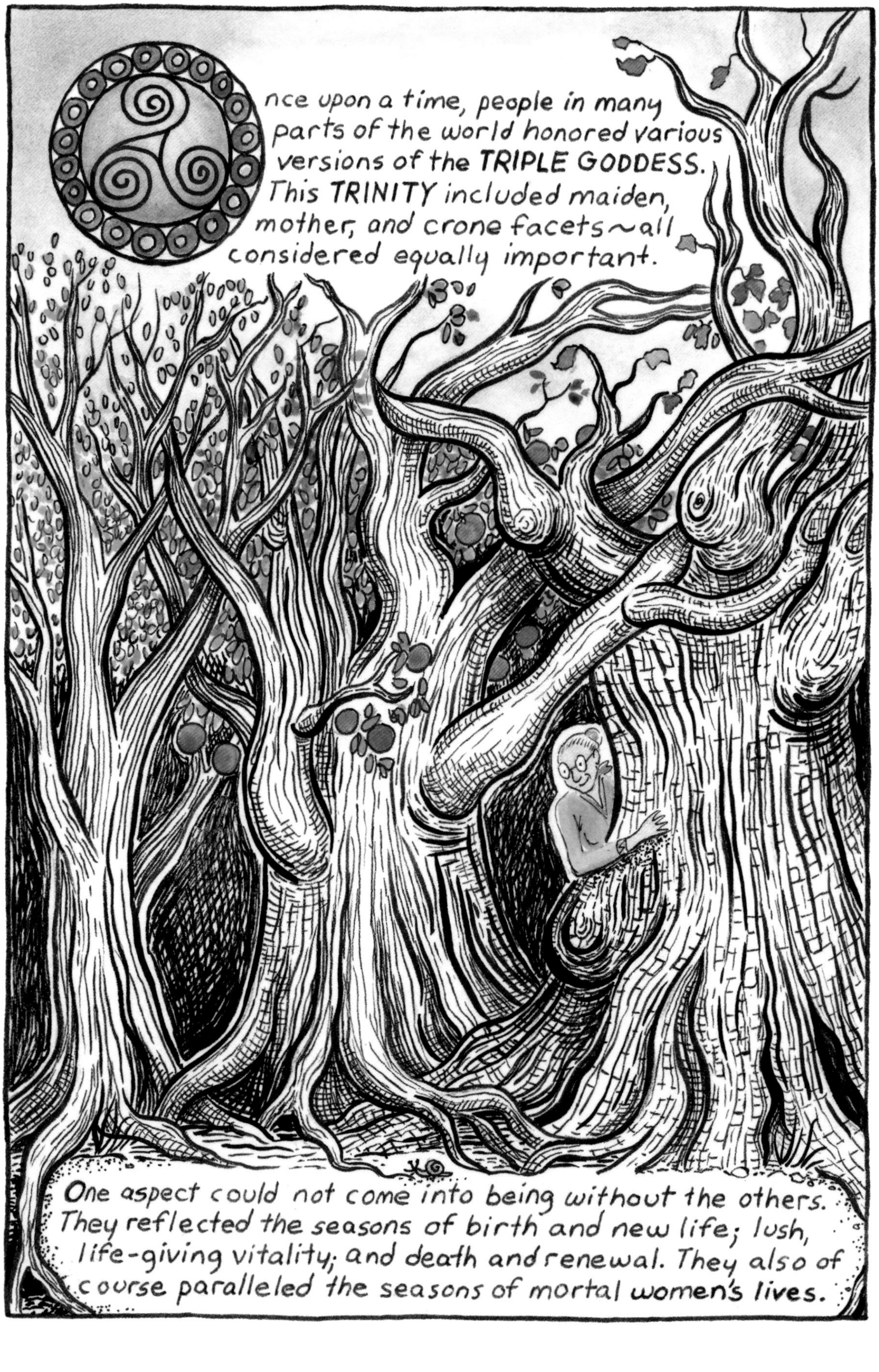
Once upon a time, people in many parts of the world honored various versions of the TRIPLE GODDESS. This TRINITY included maiden, mother, and crone facets~all considered equally important.
One aspect could not come into being without the others. They reflected the seasons of birth and new life; lush, life-giving vitality; and death and renewal. They also of course paralleled the seasons of mortal women's lives.

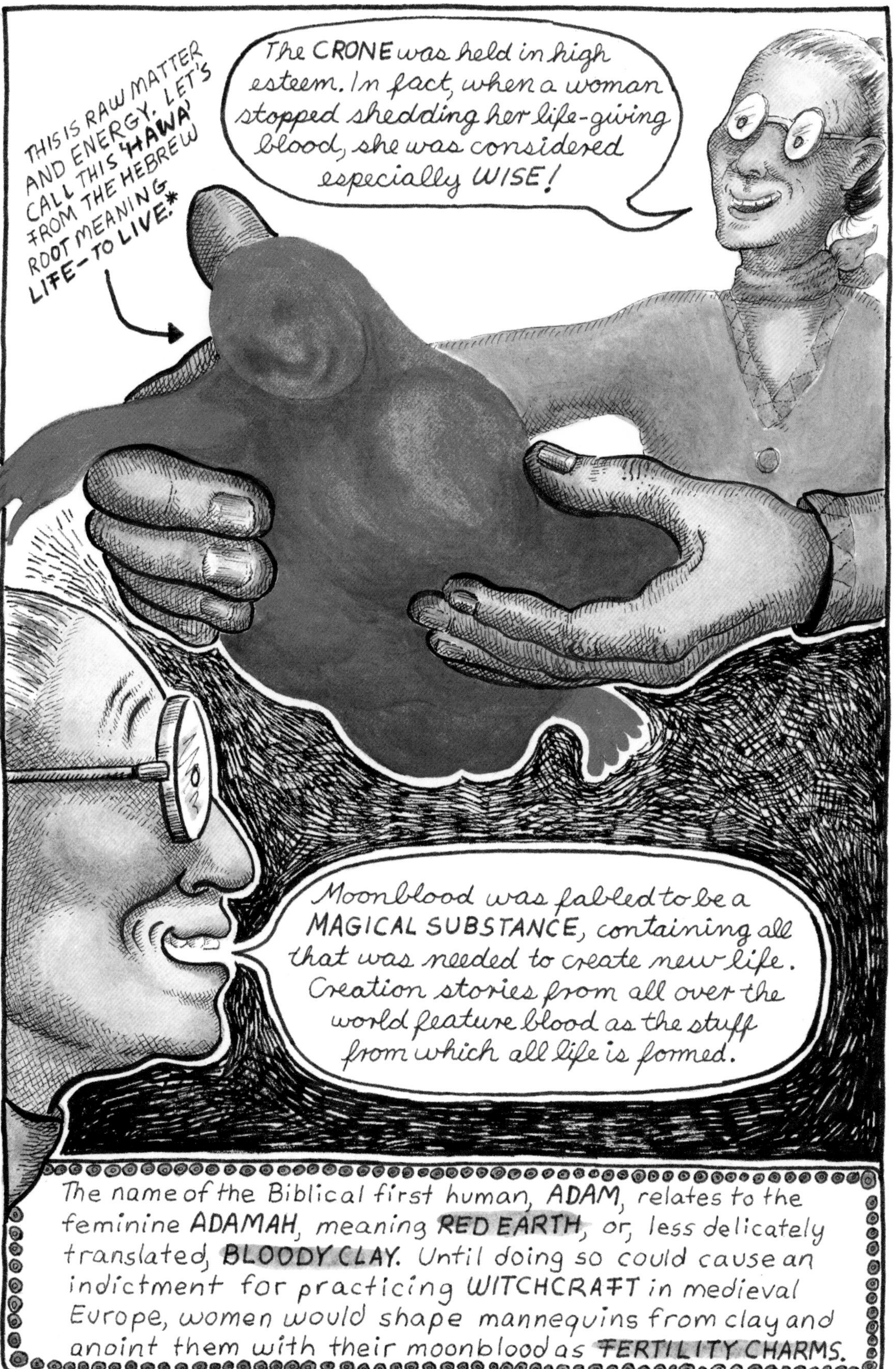
The CRONE was held in high esteem. In fact, when a woman stopped shedding her life-giving blood, she was considered especially WISE!
THIS IS RAW MATTER AND ENERGY. LET'S CALL THIS 'HAWA' FROM THE HEBREW ROOT MEANING LIFE–TO LIVE.*
Moonblood was fabled to be a MAGICAL SUBSTANCE, containing all that was needed to create new life. Creation stories from all over the world feature blood as the stuff from which all life is formed.
The name of the Biblical first human, ADAM, relates to the feminine ADAMAH, meaning RED EARTH, or, less delicately translated, BLOODY CLAY. Until doing so could cause an indictment for practicing WITCHCRAFT in medieval Europe, women would shape mannequins from clay and anoint them with their moonblood as FERTILITY CHARMS.

*HAWA IS ALSO THE ROOT OF THE NAME **EVE**.

So...when a woman stopped her menses, it meant she kept all of that vitality WITHIN. Instead of using her magical power to gestate babies, she was FREE to create ANYTHING she chose.

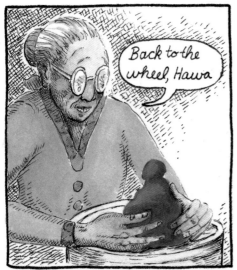

Back to the wheel, Hawa

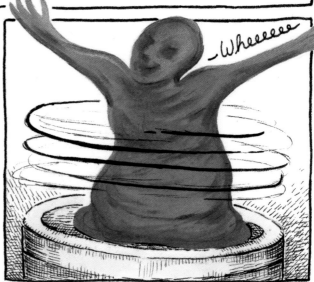

—Wheeeeee

Speaking of WHEELS, when patriarchal sensibilities took over, instead of the ever-turning wheel of life that honored seasons and life's cycles, the central image of perfection and health began to feature an idealized male. Deviations from this "norm" were pathologized. Menopause became a condition to be managed.

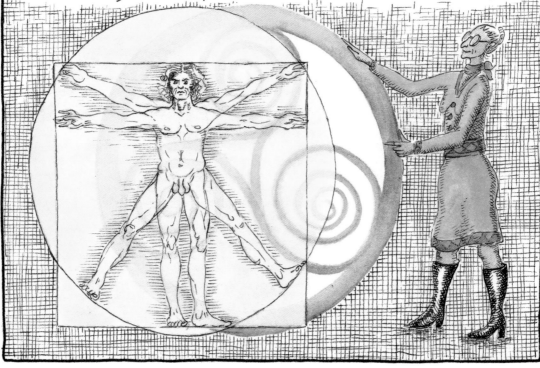

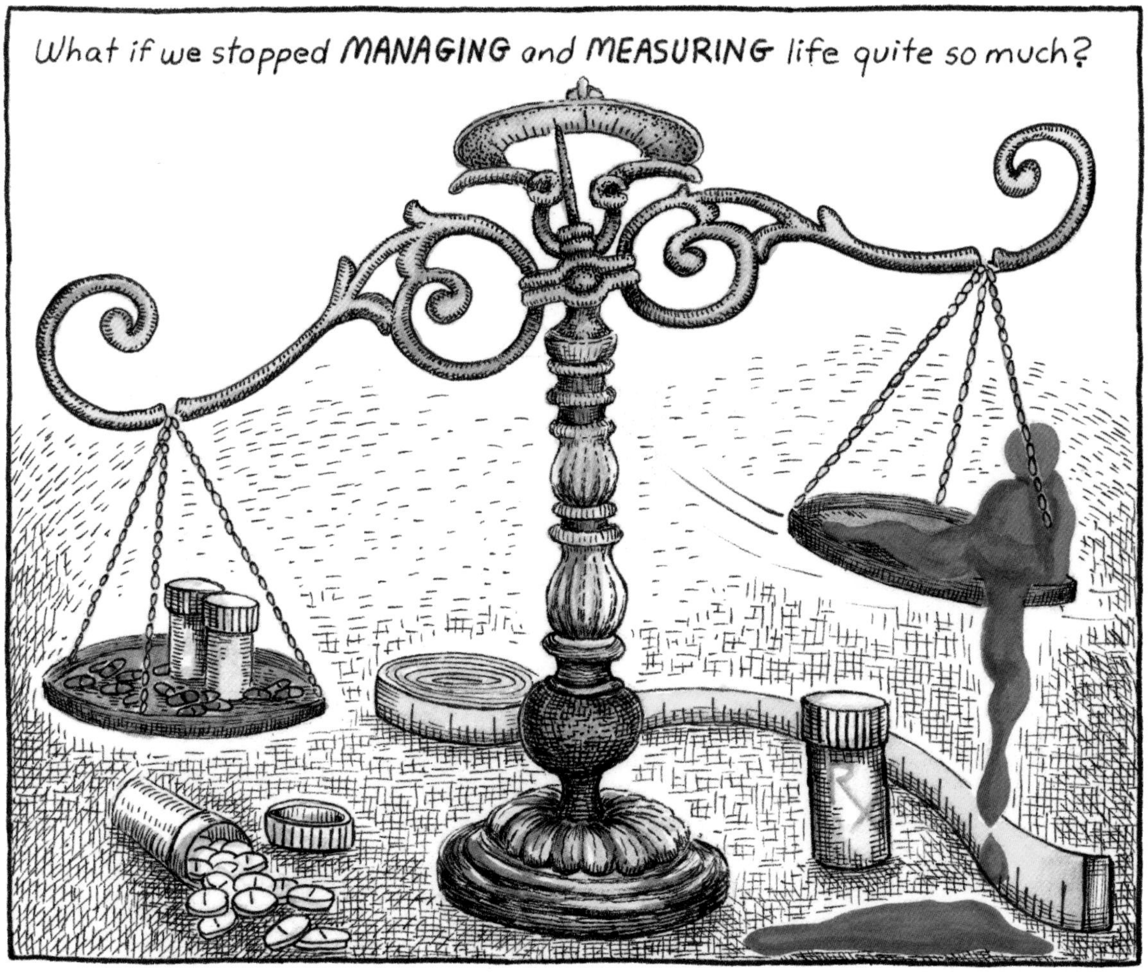
What if we stopped MANAGING and MEASURING life quite so much?
Rx

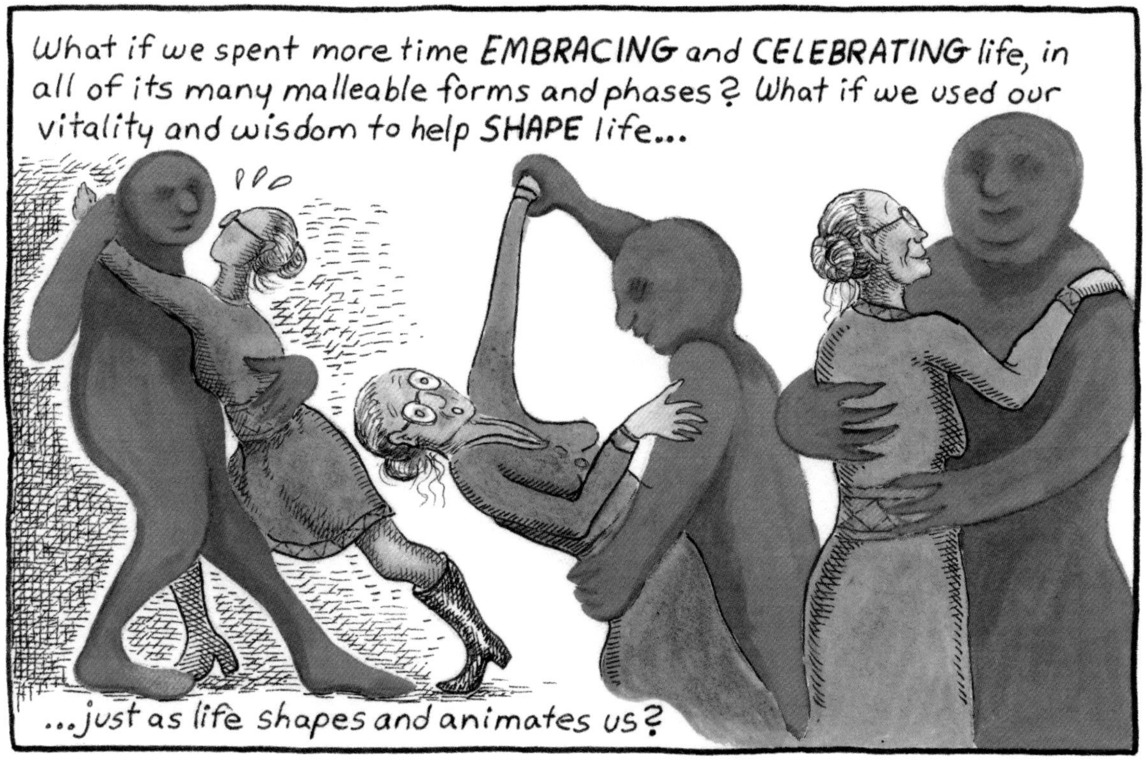
What if we spent more time EMBRACING and CELEBRATING life, in all of its many malleable forms and phases? What if we used our vitality and wisdom to help SHAPE life...
...just as life shapes and animates us?

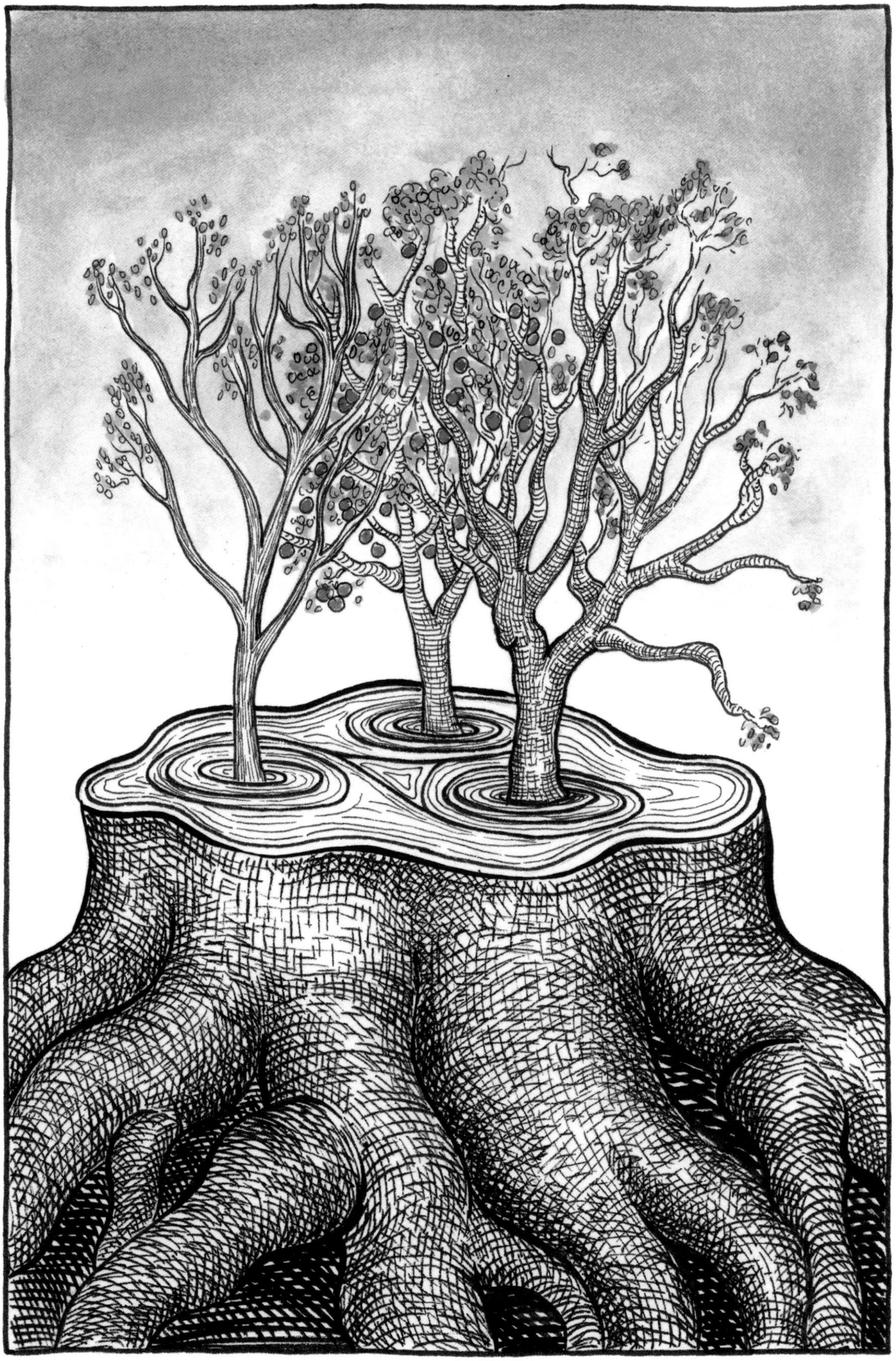

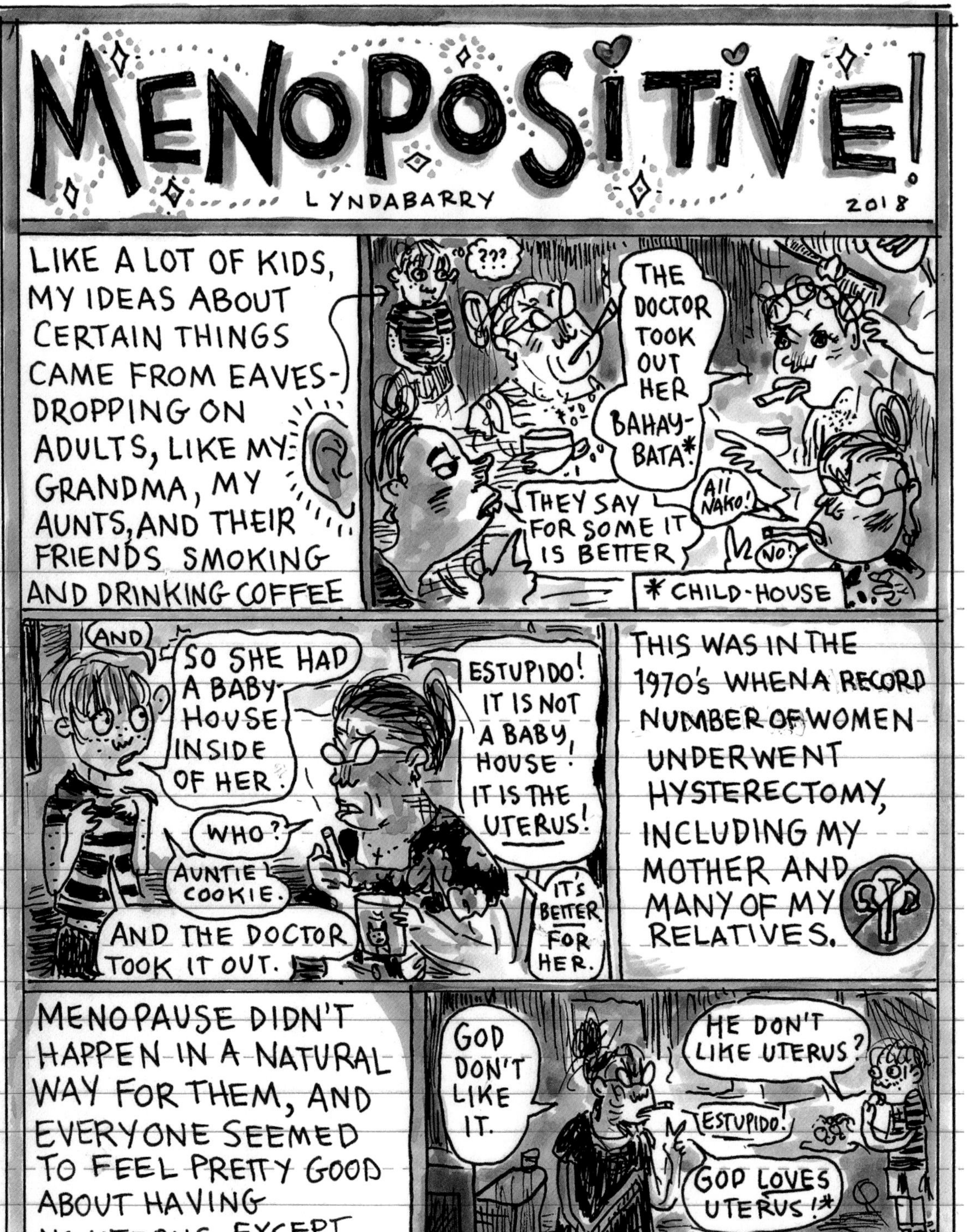
MENOPOSITIVE!
LYNDABARRY
2018
LIKE A LOT OF KIDS, MY IDEAS ABOUT CERTAIN THINGS CAME FROM EAVES-DROPPING ON ADULTS, LIKE MY GRANDMA, MY AUNTS, AND THEIR FRIENDS SMOKING AND DRINKING COFFEE
???
THE DOCTOR TOOK OUT HER BAHAY-BATA*
THEY SAY FOR SOME IT IS BETTER
AII NAKO!
NO!
* CHILD-HOUSE
AND
SO SHE HAD A BABY-HOUSE INSIDE OF HER.
WHO?
AUNTIE COOKIE.
AND THE DOCTOR TOOK IT OUT.
ESTUPIDO! IT IS NOT A BABY HOUSE! IT IS THE UTERUS!
IT'S BETTER FOR HER.
THIS WAS IN THE 1970'S WHEN A RECORD NUMBER OF WOMEN UNDERWENT HYSTERECTOMY, INCLUDING MY MOTHER AND MANY OF MY RELATIVES.
MENOPAUSE DIDN'T HAPPEN IN A NATURAL WAY FOR THEM, AND EVERYONE SEEMED TO FEEL PRETTY GOOD ABOUT HAVING NO UTERUS. EXCEPT MY GRANDMA WASN'T INTO IT, THOUGH.
GOD DON'T LIKE IT.
HE DON'T LIKE UTERUS?
ESTUPIDO!
GOD LOVES UTERUS!*
*(SOUNDS BETTER IN TAGALOG)

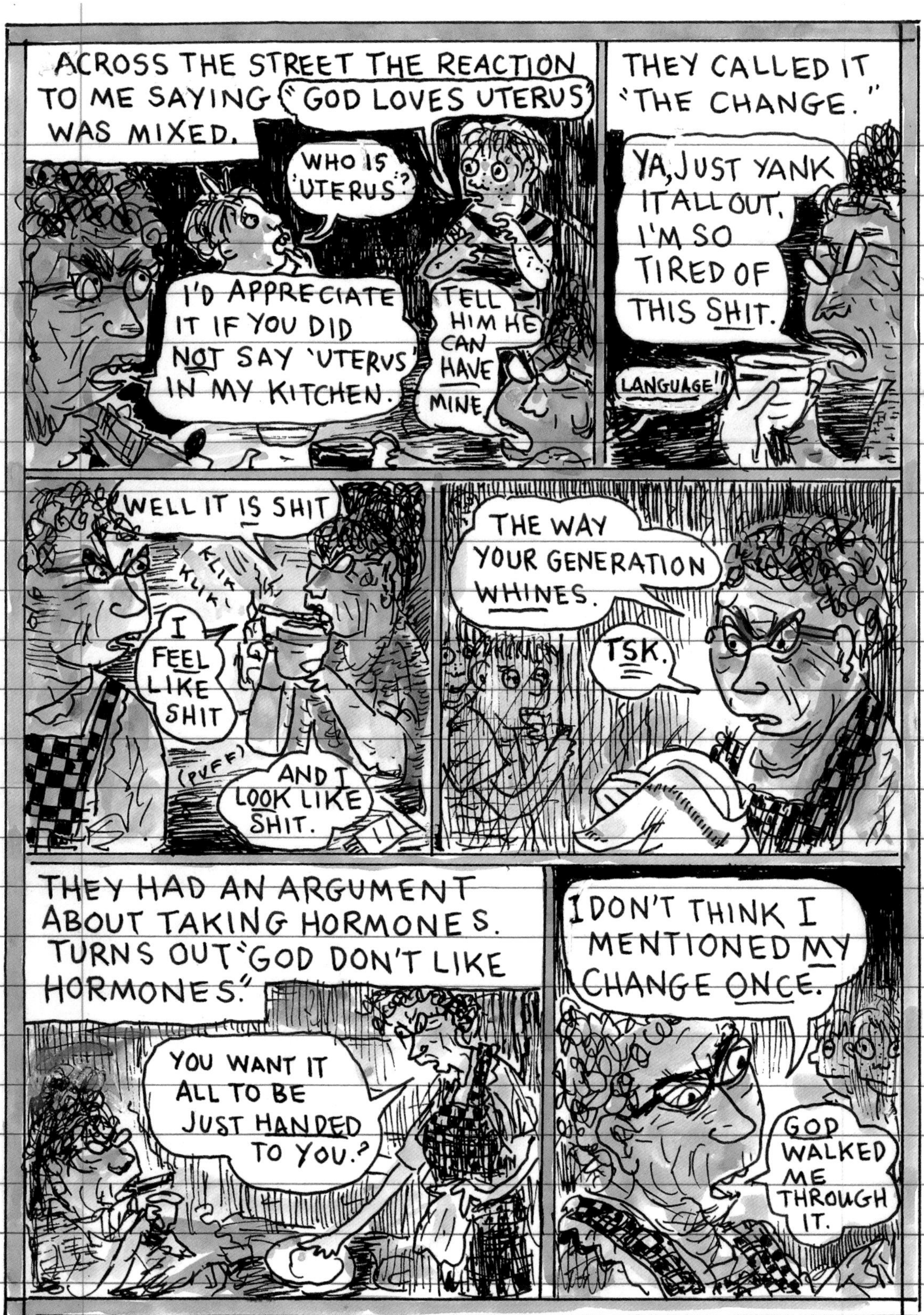
ACROSS THE STREET THE REACTION TO ME SAYING "GOD LOVES UTERUS" WAS MIXED.
WHO IS 'UTERUS'?
I'D APPRECIATE IT IF YOU DID NOT SAY 'UTERUS' IN MY KITCHEN.
TELL HIM HE CAN HAVE MINE
THEY CALLED IT "THE CHANGE."
YA, JUST YANK IT ALL OUT. I'M SO TIRED OF THIS SHIT.
LANGUAGE!
WELL IT IS SHIT
KLIK KLIK
I FEEL LIKE SHIT
(PUFF)
AND I LOOK LIKE SHIT.
THE WAY YOUR GENERATION WHINES.
TSK.
THEY HAD AN ARGUMENT ABOUT TAKING HORMONES. TURNS OUT "GOD DON'T LIKE HORMONES."
YOU WANT IT ALL TO BE JUST HANDED TO YOU.
I DON'T THINK I MENTIONED MY CHANGE ONCE.
GOD WALKED ME THROUGH IT.

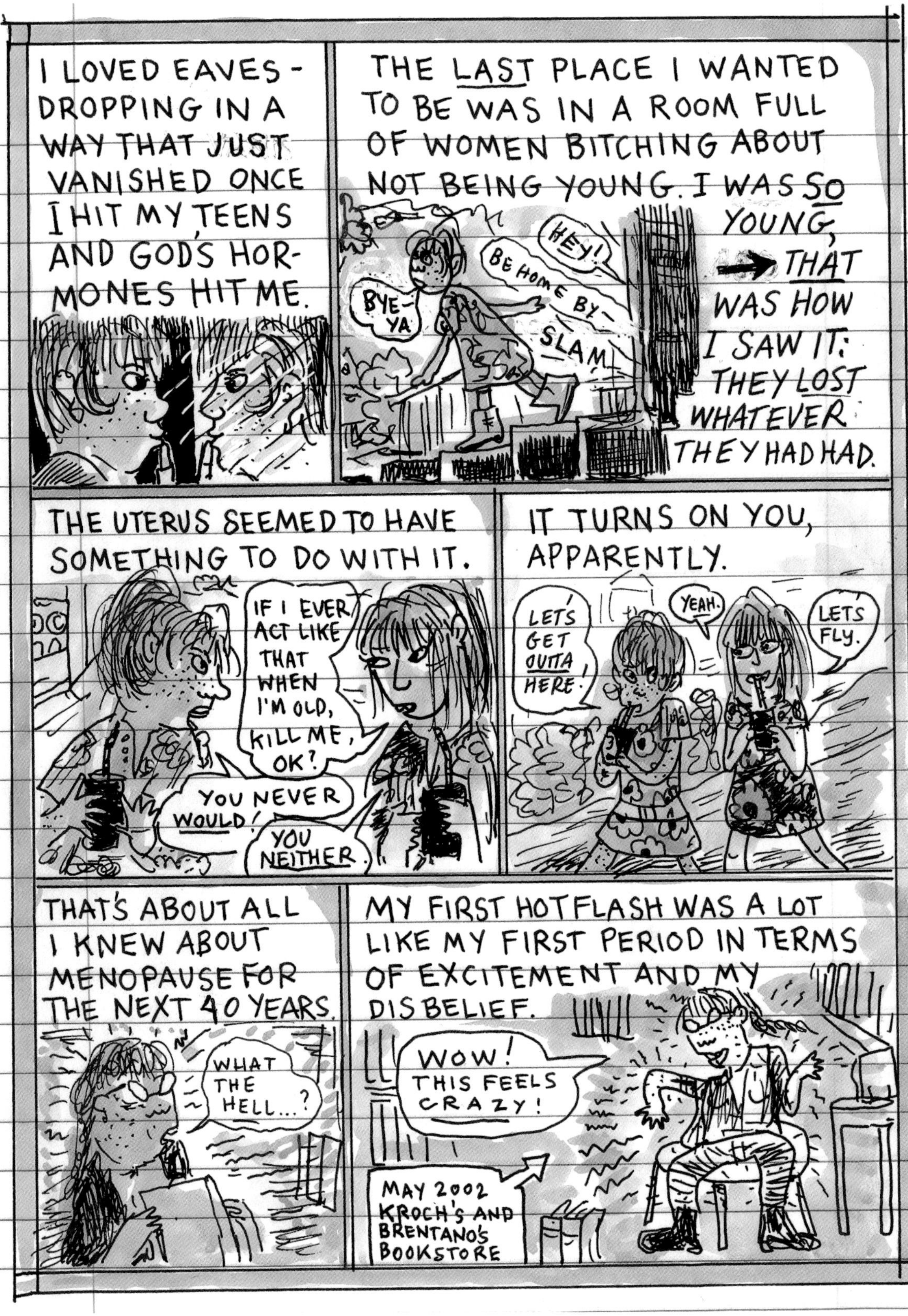
I LOVED EAVES-DROPPING IN A WAY THAT JUST VANISHED ONCE I HIT MY TEENS AND GOD'S HORMONES HIT ME.
THE LAST PLACE I WANTED TO BE WAS IN A ROOM FULL OF WOMEN BITCHING ABOUT NOT BEING YOUNG. I WAS SO YOUNG,
HEY!
BE HOME BY-
BYE-YA
SLAM
→ THAT WAS HOW I SAW IT: THEY LOST WHATEVER THEY HAD HAD.
THE UTERUS SEEMED TO HAVE SOMETHING TO DO WITH IT.
IF I EVER ACT LIKE THAT WHEN I'M OLD, KILL ME, OK?
YOU NEVER WOULD!
YOU NEITHER.
IT TURNS ON YOU, APPARENTLY.
LET'S GET OUTTA HERE!
YEAH.
LETS FLY.
THAT'S ABOUT ALL I KNEW ABOUT MENOPAUSE FOR THE NEXT 40 YEARS.
WHAT THE HELL...?
MY FIRST HOTFLASH WAS A LOT LIKE MY FIRST PERIOD IN TERMS OF EXCITEMENT AND MY DISBELIEF.
WOW! THIS FEELS CRAZY!
MAY 2002 KROCH'S AND BRENTANO'S BOOKSTORE

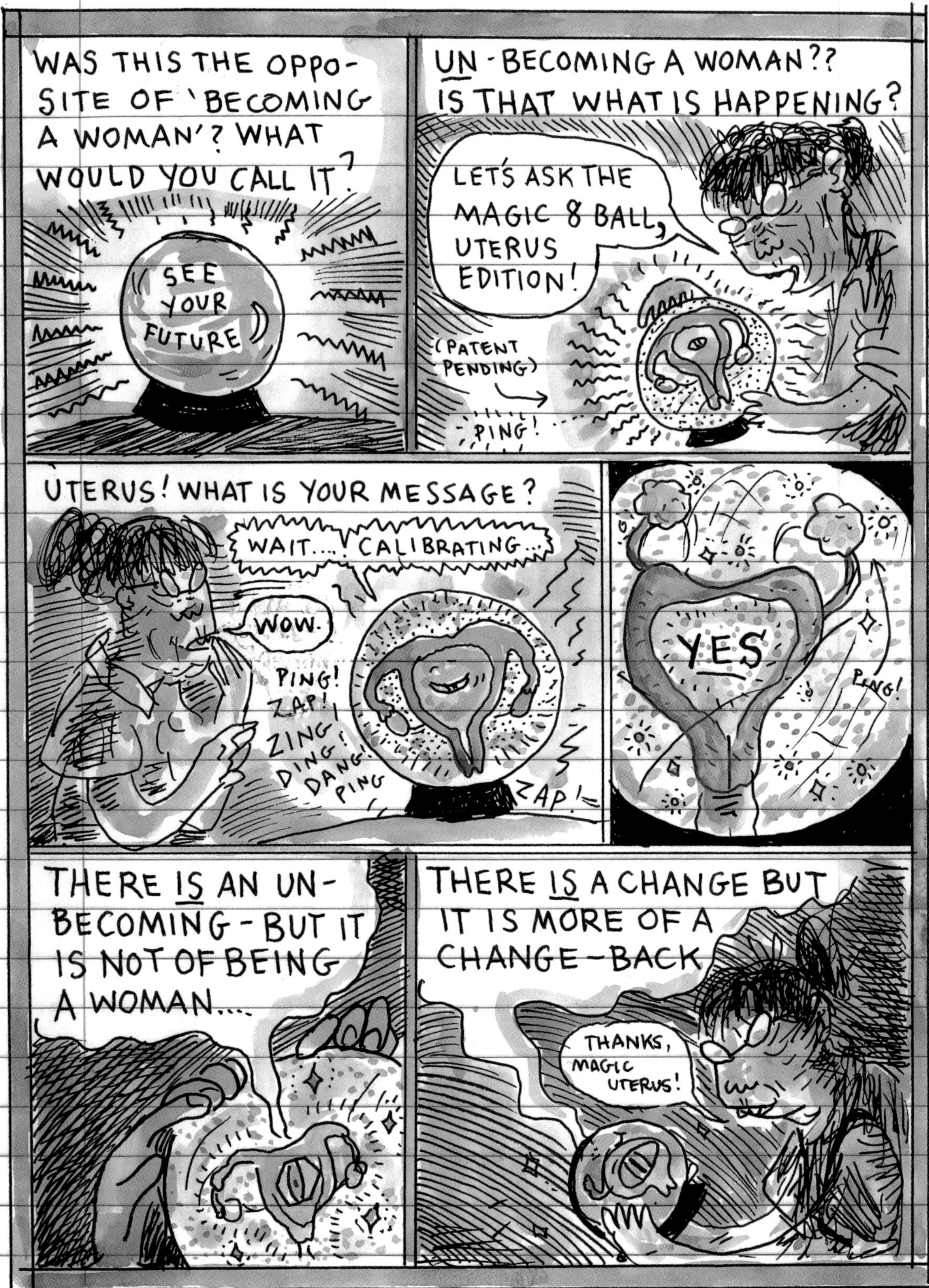
WAS THIS THE OPPOSITE OF 'BECOMING A WOMAN'? WHAT WOULD YOU CALL IT?
SEE YOUR FUTURE
UN-BECOMING A WOMAN?? IS THAT WHAT IS HAPPENING?
LET'S ASK THE MAGIC 8 BALL, UTERUS EDITION!
(PATENT PENDING)
PING!
UTERUS! WHAT IS YOUR MESSAGE?
WAIT.... CALIBRATING....
WOW.
PING! ZAP! ZING! DING! DANG! PING
ZAP!
YES
PING!
THERE IS AN UN-BECOMING - BUT IT IS NOT OF BEING A WOMAN....
THERE IS A CHANGE BUT IT IS MORE OF A CHANGE-BACK
THANKS, MAGIC UTERUS!

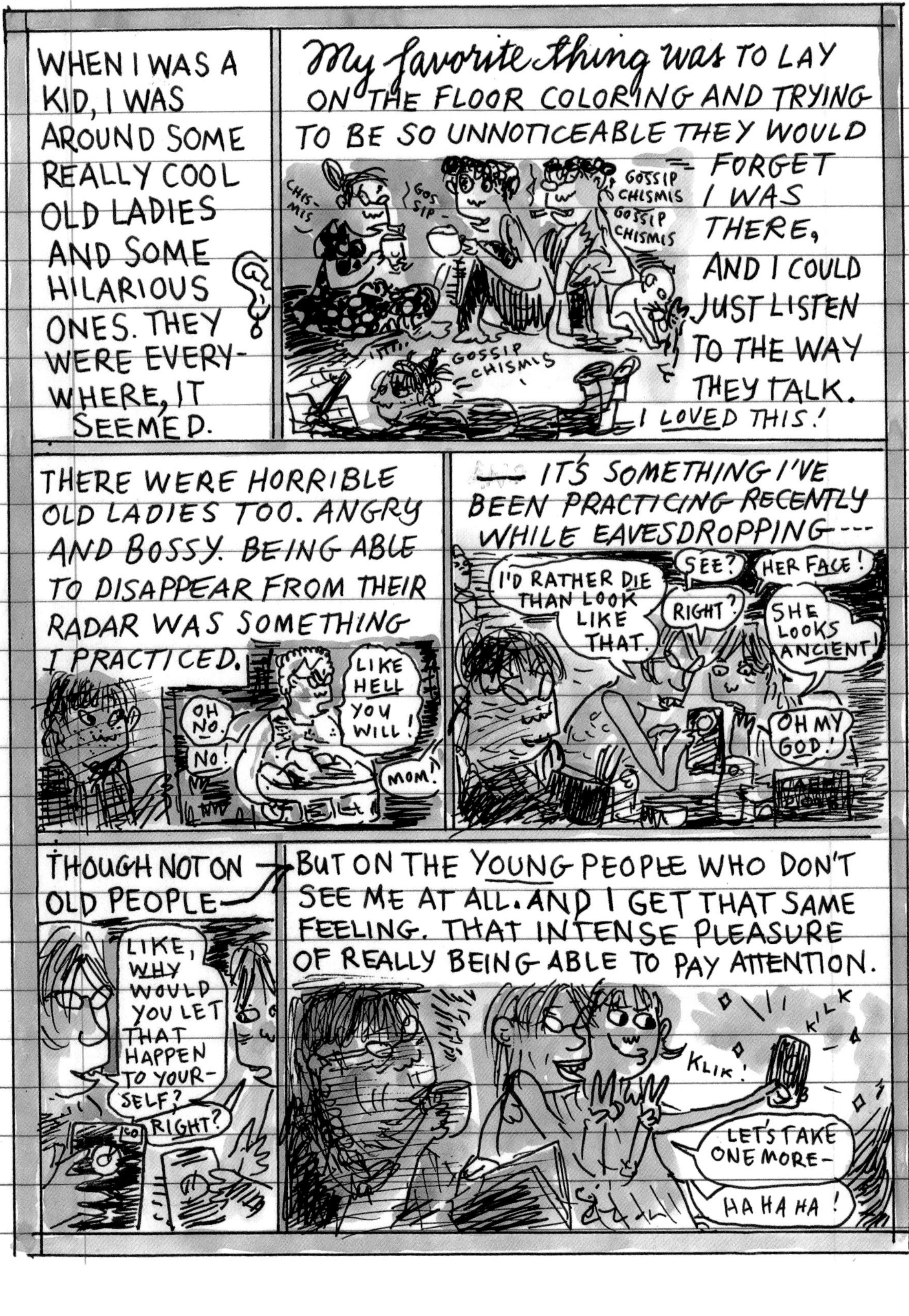
WHEN I WAS A KID, I WAS AROUND SOME REALLY COOL OLD LADIES AND SOME HILARIOUS ONES. THEY WERE EVERY-WHERE, IT SEEMED.
My favorite thing was TO LAY ON THE FLOOR COLORING AND TRYING TO BE SO UNNOTICEABLE THEY WOULD FORGET I WAS THERE, AND I COULD JUST LISTEN TO THE WAY THEY TALK.
CHIS-MIS
GOS-SIP
GOSSIP CHISMIS
GOSSIP CHISMIS
GOSSIP CHISMIS
I LOVED THIS!
THERE WERE HORRIBLE OLD LADIES TOO. ANGRY AND BOSSY. BEING ABLE TO DISAPPEAR FROM THEIR RADAR WAS SOMETHING I PRACTICED.
OH NO.
NO!
LIKE HELL YOU WILL!
MOM!
— IT'S SOMETHING I'VE BEEN PRACTICING RECENTLY WHILE EAVESDROPPING---
I'D RATHER DIE THAN LOOK LIKE THAT.
SEE?
RIGHT?
HER FACE!
SHE LOOKS ANCIENT!
OH MY GOD!
THOUGH NOT ON OLD PEOPLE—
LIKE, WHY WOULD YOU LET THAT HAPPEN TO YOUR-SELF?
RIGHT?
BUT ON THE YOUNG PEOPLE WHO DON'T SEE ME AT ALL. AND I GET THAT SAME FEELING. THAT INTENSE PLEASURE OF REALLY BEING ABLE TO PAY ATTENTION.
KLIK!
KLIK
LET'S TAKE ONE MORE—
HA HA HA!

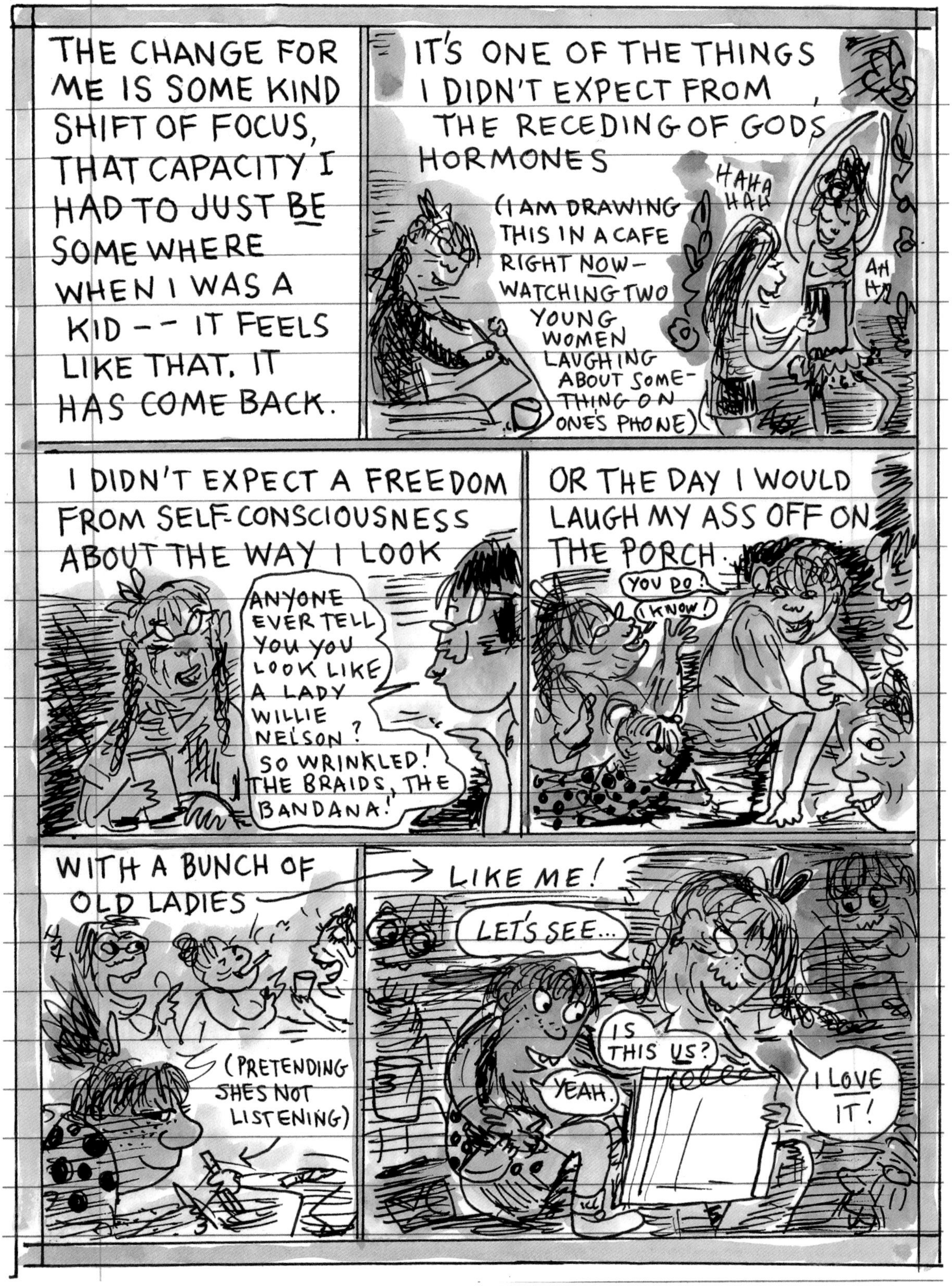
THE CHANGE FOR ME IS SOME KIND SHIFT OF FOCUS, THAT CAPACITY I HAD TO JUST BE SOME WHERE WHEN I WAS A KID -- IT FEELS LIKE THAT. IT HAS COME BACK.
IT'S ONE OF THE THINGS I DIDN'T EXPECT FROM THE RECEDING OF GODS HORMONES
(I AM DRAWING THIS IN A CAFE RIGHT NOW- WATCHING TWO YOUNG WOMEN LAUGHING ABOUT SOMETHING ON ONE'S PHONE)
HAHA HAH
AH HA
I DIDN'T EXPECT A FREEDOM FROM SELF-CONSCIOUSNESS ABOUT THE WAY I LOOK
ANYONE EVER TELL YOU YOU LOOK LIKE A LADY WILLIE NELSON?
SO WRINKLED! THE BRAIDS, THE BANDANA!
OR THE DAY I WOULD LAUGH MY ASS OFF ON THE PORCH.
YOU DO!
I KNOW!
WITH A BUNCH OF OLD LADIES
LIKE ME!
(PRETENDING SHES NOT LISTENING)
LET'S SEE...
IS THIS US?
YEAH.
I LOVE IT!

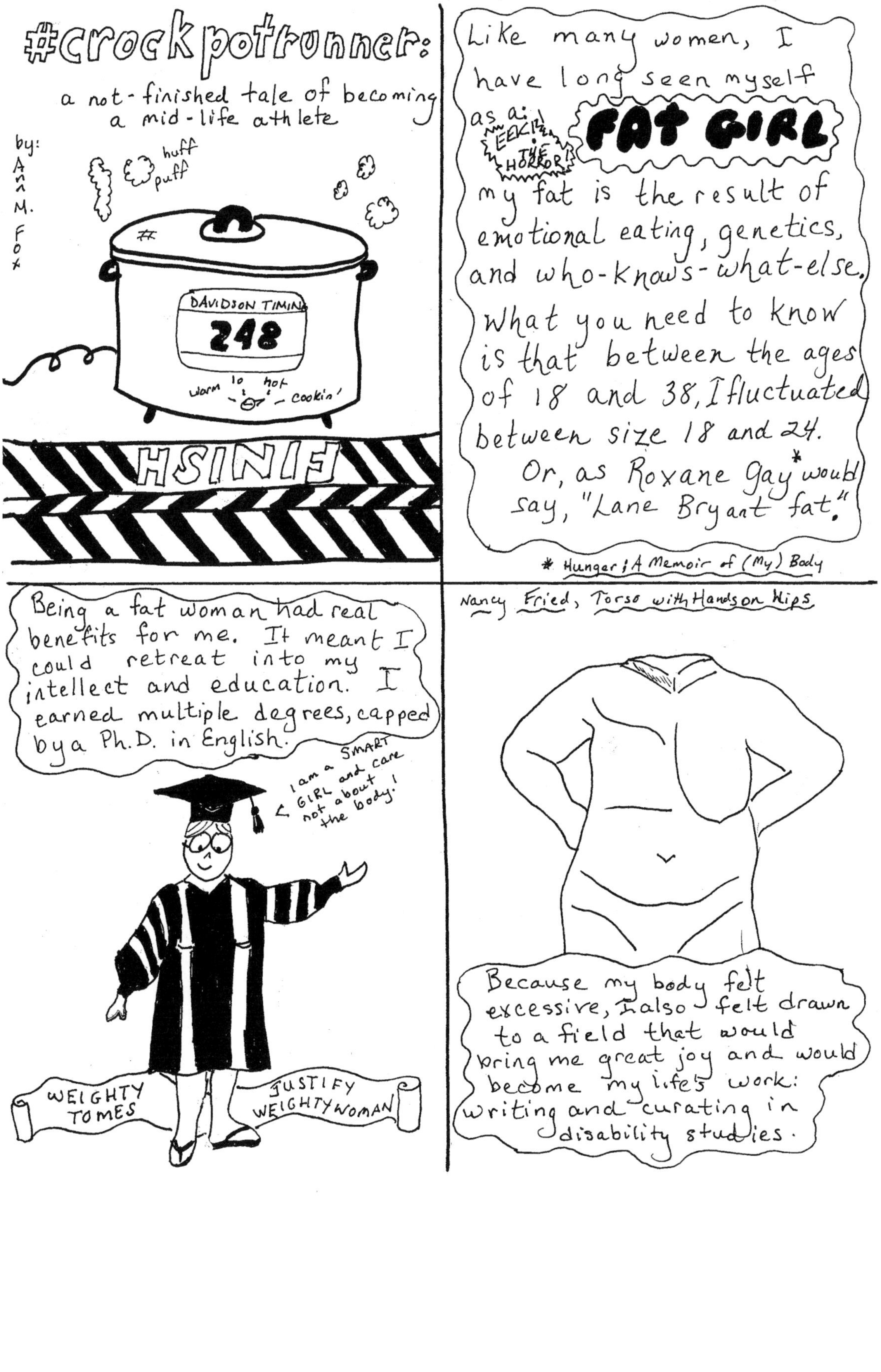
#crockpotrunner:
a not-finished tale of becoming a mid-life athlete
by: Ann M. Fox
huff puff
#
DAVIDSON TIMING
248
warm lo hot
cookin'
FINISH
Like many women, I have long seen myself as a:
EEK!! THE HORROR!
FAT GIRL
my fat is the result of emotional eating, genetics, and who-knows-what-else.
What you need to know is that between the ages of 18 and 38, I fluctuated between size 18 and 24.
Or, as Roxane Gay* would say, "Lane Bryant fat."
* Hunger: A Memoir of (My) Body
Being a fat woman had real benefits for me. It meant I could retreat into my intellect and education. I earned multiple degrees, capped by a Ph.D. in English.
I am a SMART GIRL and care not about the body!
WEIGHTY TOMES
JUSTIFY WEIGHTY WOMAN
Nancy Fried, Torso with Hands on Hips
Because my body felt excessive, I also felt drawn to a field that would bring me great joy and would become my life's work: writing and curating in disability studies.

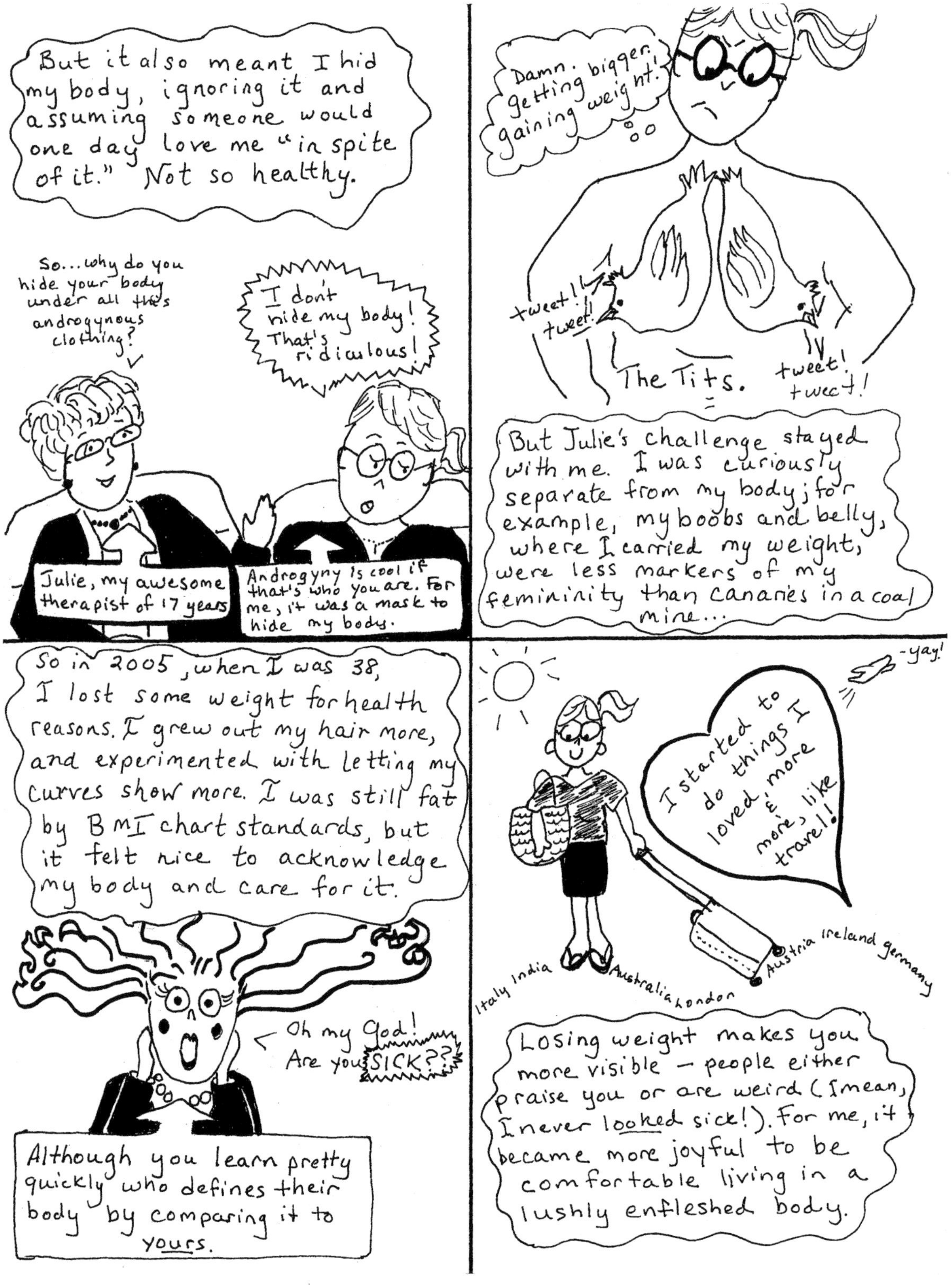

But it also meant I hid my body, ignoring it and assuming someone would one day love me "in spite of it." Not so healthy.
Damn. bigger. getting gaining weight!
tweet! tweet!
The Tits.
tweet! tweet!
But Julie's challenge stayed with me. I was curiously separate from my body; for example, my boobs and belly, where I carried my weight, were less markers of my femininity than canaries in a coal mine...
So... why do you hide your body under all this androgynous clothing?
I don't hide my body! That's ridiculous!
Julie, my awesome therapist of 17 years
Androgyny is cool if that's who you are. For me, it was a mask to hide my body.
So in 2005, when I was 38, I lost some weight for health reasons. I grew out my hair more, and experimented with letting my curves show more. I was still fat by BMI chart standards, but it felt nice to acknowledge my body and care for it.
Oh my God! Are you SICK??
Although you learn pretty quickly who defines their body by comparing it to yours.
-yay!
I started to do things I loved, more & more, like travel!
Italy India Australia London Austria Ireland Germany
Losing weight makes you more visible – people either praise you or are weird (I mean, I never looked sick!). For me, it became more joyful to be comfortable living in a lushly enfleshed body.

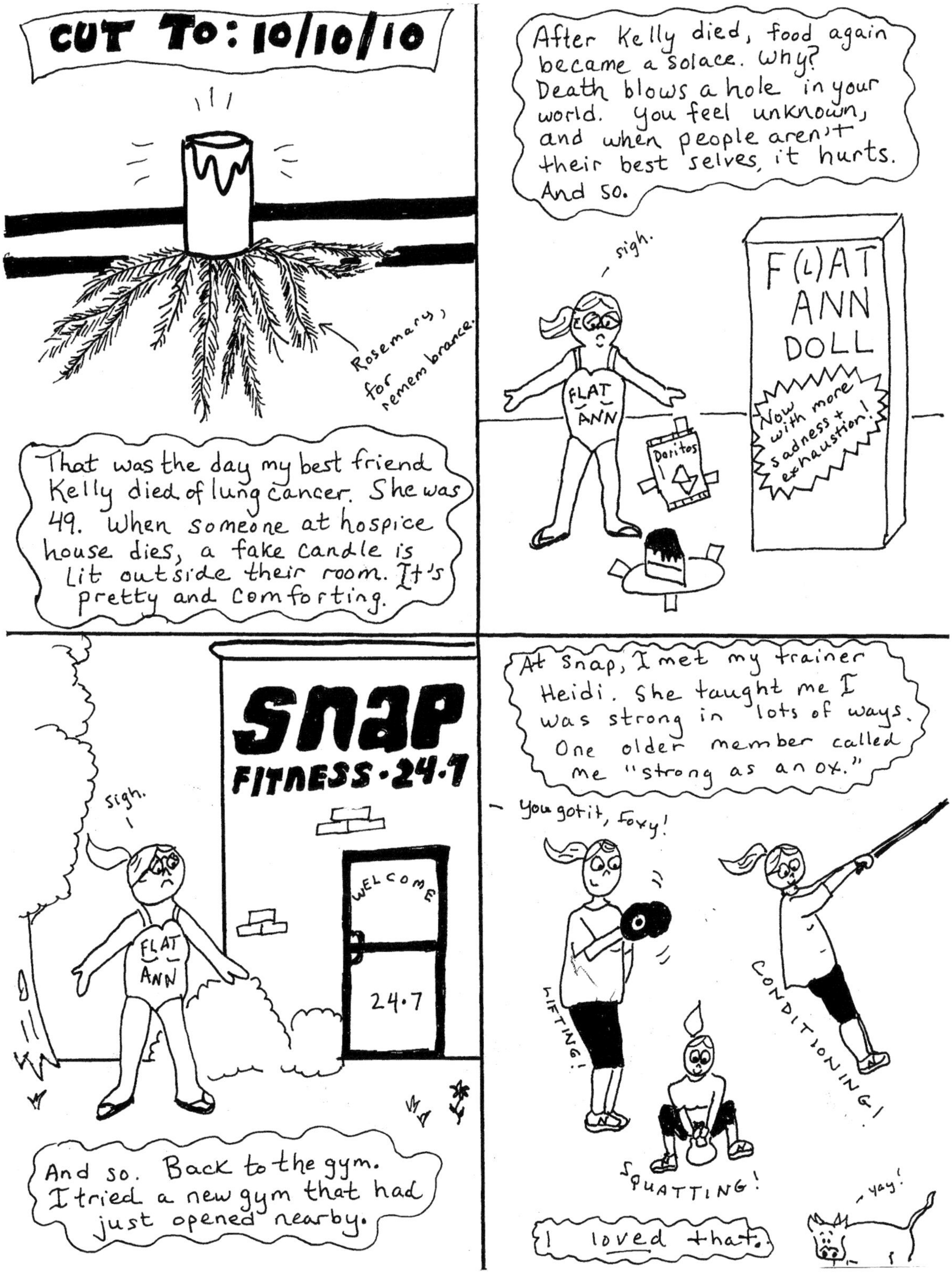
CUT TO: 10/10/10
Rosemary, for remembrance.
That was the day my best friend Kelly died of lung cancer. She was 49. When someone at hospice house dies, a fake candle is lit outside their room. It's pretty and comforting.
After Kelly died, food again became a solace. Why? Death blows a hole in your world. You feel unknown, and when people aren't their best selves, it hurts. And so.
sigh.
FLAT ANN
Doritos
F(L)AT ANN DOLL
Now with more sadness + exhaustion!
SNAP FITNESS • 24•7
sigh.
FLAT ANN
WELCOME
24•7
And so. Back to the gym. I tried a new gym that had just opened nearby.
At Snap, I met my trainer Heidi. She taught me I was strong in lots of ways. One older member called me "strong as an ox."
You got it, Foxy!
LIFTING!
CONDITIONING!
SQUATTING!
yay!
I loved that.

#crockpotrunner

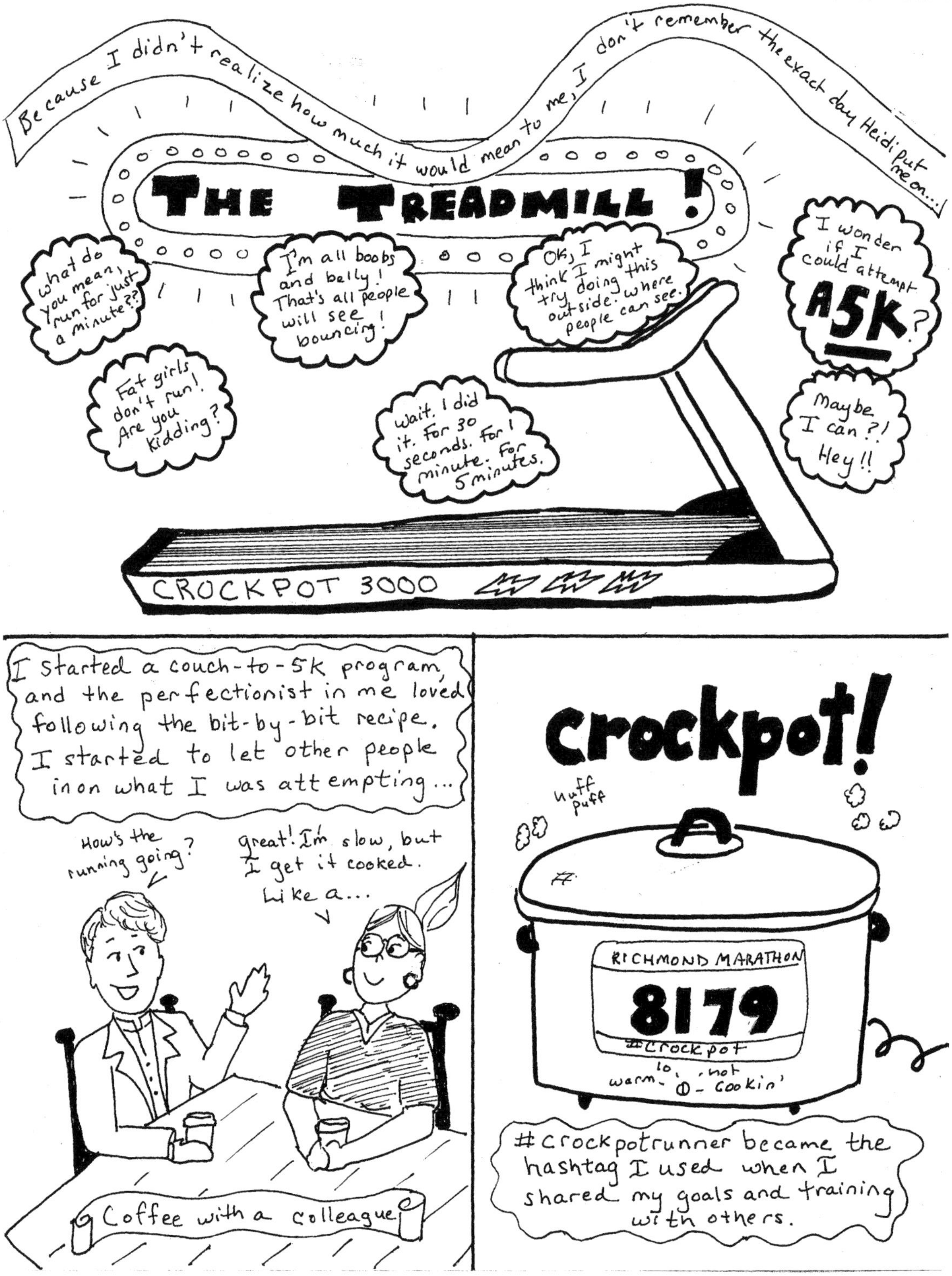
Because I didn't realize how much it would mean to me, I don't remember the exact day Heidi put me on...
THE TREADMILL!
What do you mean, run for just a minute??
Fat girls don't run! Are you kidding?
I'm all boobs and belly! That's all people will see bouncing!
Wait. I did it. For 30 seconds. For 1 minute. For 5 minutes.
Ok, I think I might try doing this outside. where people can see.
I wonder if I could attempt A 5K?
Maybe I can?! Hey!!
CROCKPOT 3000
I started a couch-to-5k program, and the perfectionist in me loved following the bit-by-bit recipe. I started to let other people in on what I was attempting...
How's the running going?
Great! I'm slow, but I get it cooked. Like a...
Coffee with a colleague
Crockpot!
huff puff
RICHMOND MARATHON
8179
#crockpot
warm lo hot cookin'
#crockpotrunner became the hashtag I used when I shared my goals and training with others.

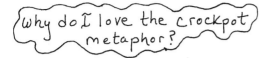

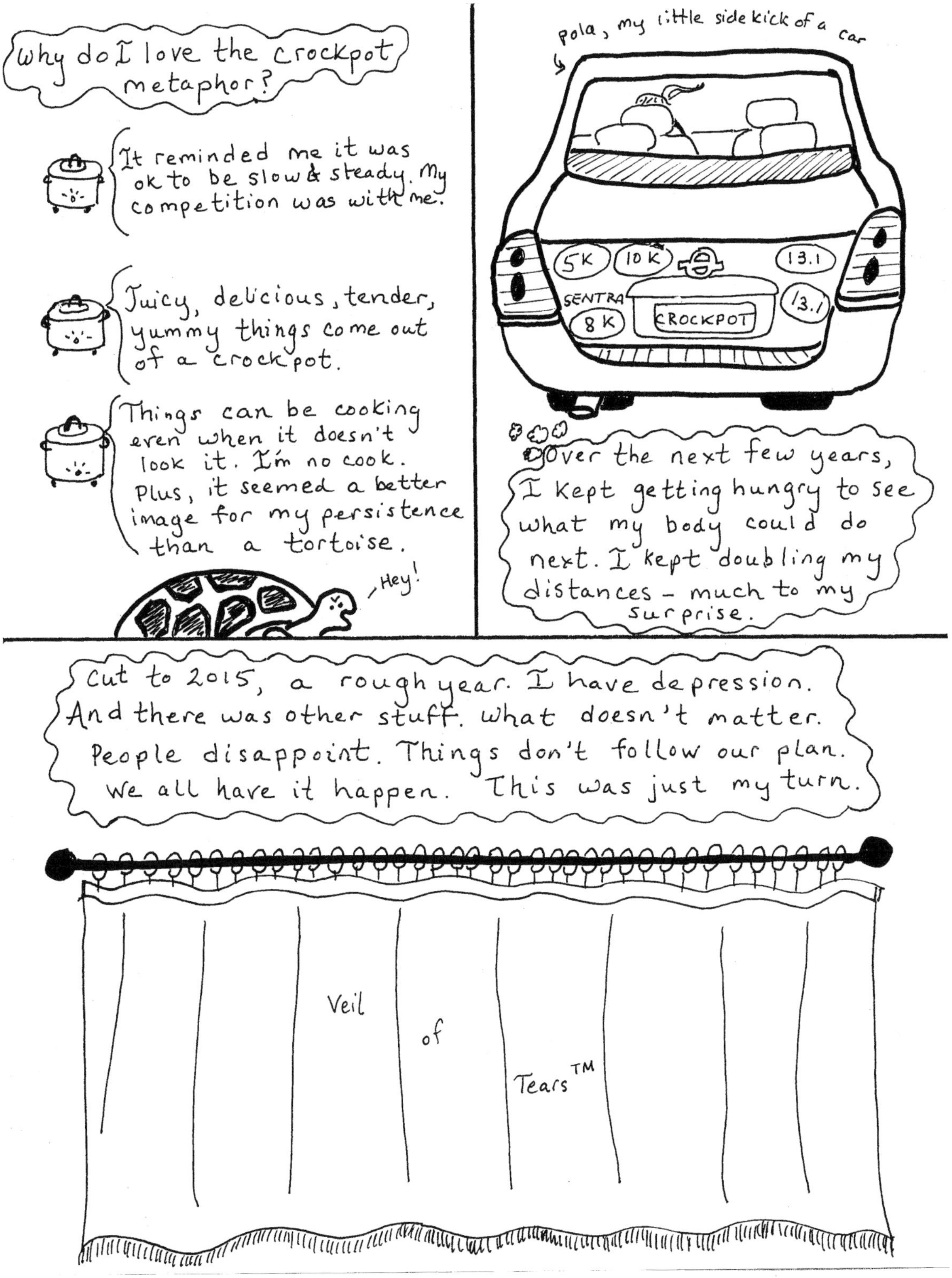

Why do I love the crockpot metaphor?

It reminded me it was ok to be slow & steady. My competition was with me.

Juicy, delicious, tender, yummy things come out of a crockpot.

Things can be cooking even when it doesn't look it. I'm no cook. Plus, it seemed a better image for my persistence than a tortoise.

Hey!

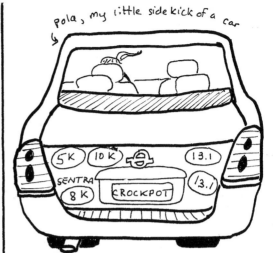

Pola, my little side kick of a car

5K 10K 13.1
SENTRA 13.1
8K CROCKPOT

Over the next few years, I kept getting hungry to see what my body could do next. I kept doubling my distances - much to my surprise.

Cut to 2015, a rough year. I have depression. And there was other stuff. What doesn't matter. People disappoint. Things don't follow our plan. We all have it happen. This was just my turn.

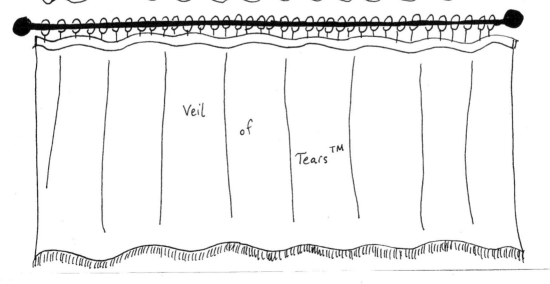

Veil of Tears™

#crockpotrunner

Ann M. Fox

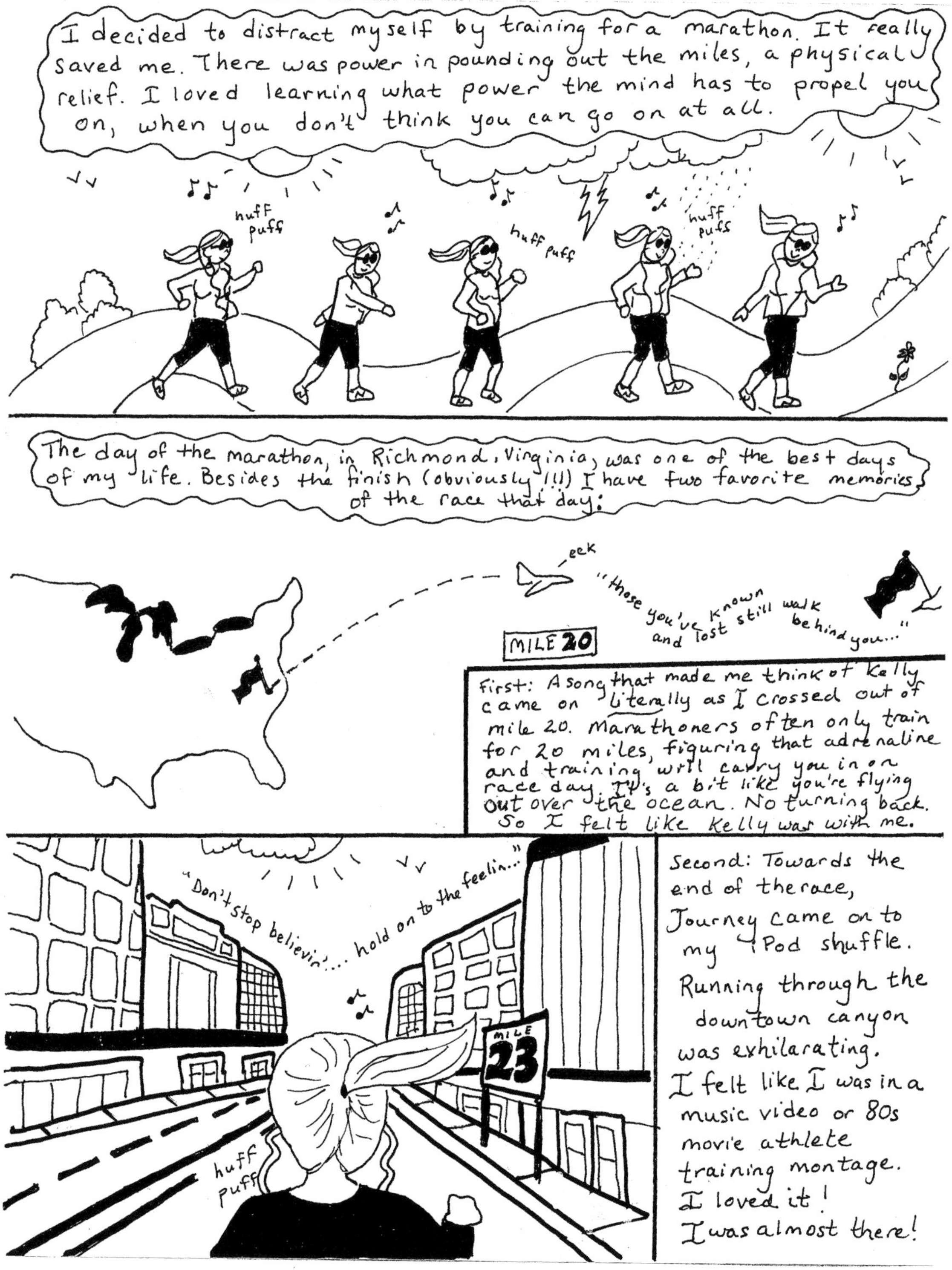
I decided to distract myself by training for a marathon. It really saved me. There was power in pounding out the miles, a physical relief. I loved learning what power the mind has to propel you on, when you don't think you can go on at all.
huff puff
huff puff
huff puffs
The day of the marathon, in Richmond, Virginia, was one of the best days of my life. Besides the finish (obviously!!!) I have two favorite memories of the race that day:
eek
"those you've known and lost still walk behind you..."
MILE 20
First: A song that made me think of Kelly came on literally as I crossed out of mile 20. Marathoners often only train for 20 miles, figuring that adrenaline and training will carry you in on race day. It's a bit like you're flying out over the ocean. No turning back. So I felt like Kelly was with me.
"Don't stop believin'... hold on to the feelin..."
MILE 23
huff puff
Second: Towards the end of the race, Journey came on to my iPod shuffle. Running through the downtown canyon was exhilarating. I felt like I was in a music video or 80s movie athlete training montage. I loved it! I was almost there!

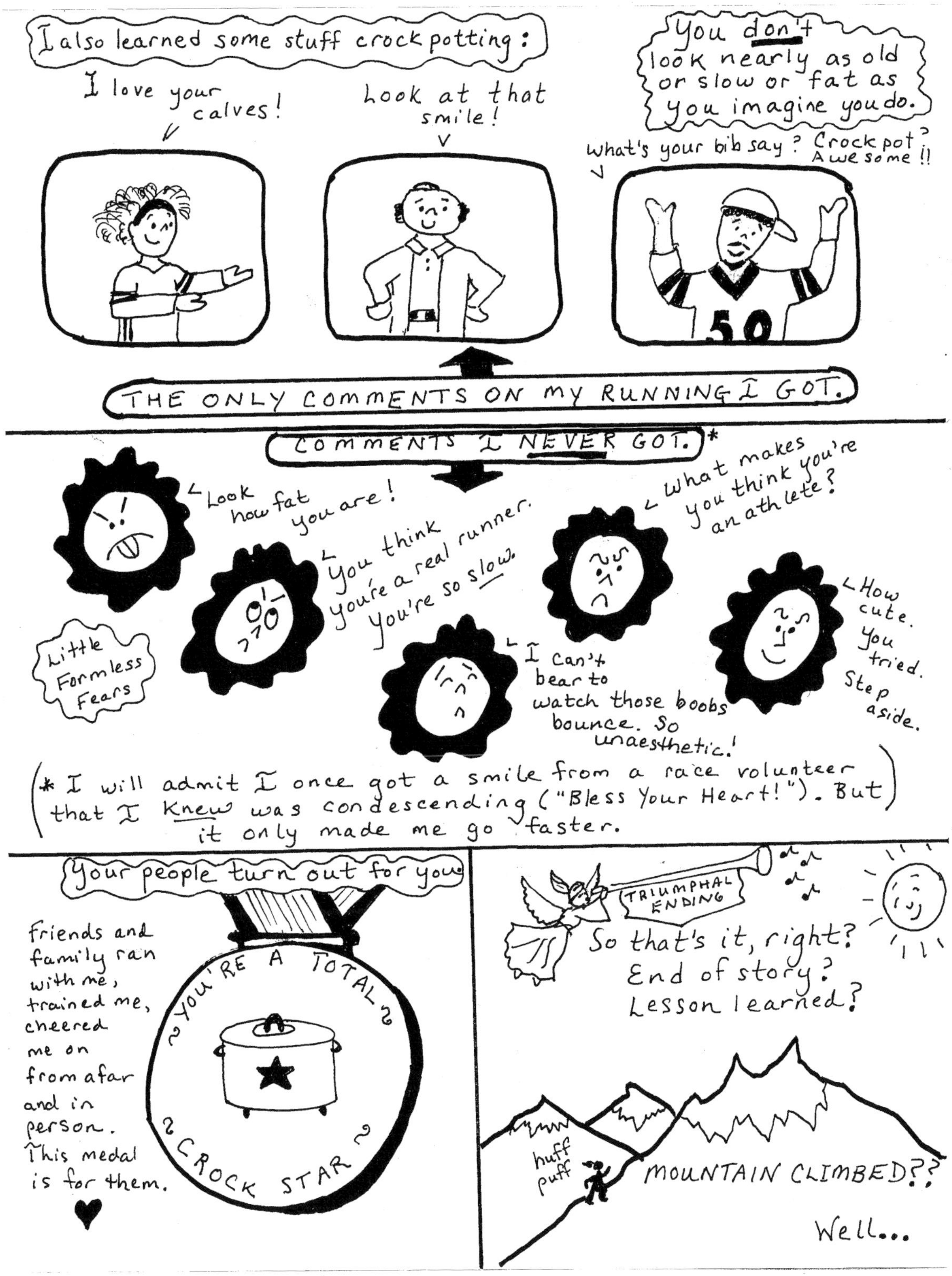

I also learned some stuff crockpotting:
I love your calves!
Look at that smile!
You don't look nearly as old or slow or fat as you imagine you do.
What's your bib say? Crockpot? Awesome!!
50
THE ONLY COMMENTS ON MY RUNNING I GOT.
COMMENTS I NEVER GOT.*
Look how fat you are!
You think you're a real runner. You're so slow.
What makes you think you're an athlete?
How cute. You tried. Step aside.
I can't bear to watch those boobs bounce. So unaesthetic!
Little Formless Fears
(* I will admit I once got a smile from a race volunteer that I knew was condescending ("Bless Your Heart!"). But it only made me go faster.
Your people turn out for you
Friends and family ran with me, trained me, cheered me on from afar and in person. This medal is for them.
YOU'RE A TOTAL CROCK STAR
TRIUMPHAL ENDING
So that's it, right? End of story? Lesson learned?
huff puff
MOUNTAIN CLIMBED??
Well...

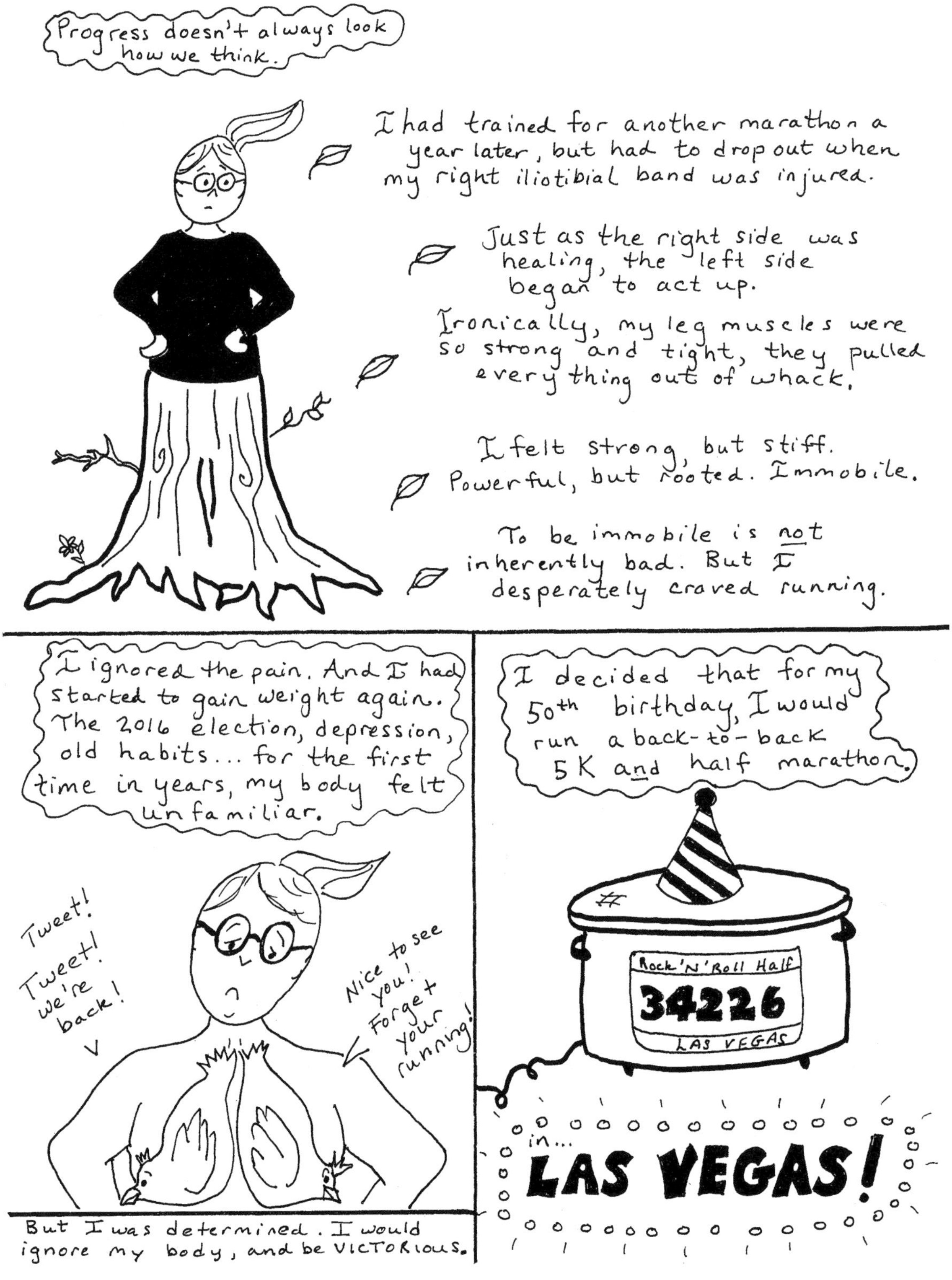
Progress doesn't always look how we think.
I had trained for another marathon a year later, but had to drop out when my right iliotibial band was injured.
Just as the right side was healing, the left side began to act up.
Ironically, my leg muscles were so strong and tight, they pulled everything out of whack.
I felt strong, but stiff. Powerful, but rooted. Immobile.
To be immobile is not inherently bad. But I desperately craved running.
I ignored the pain. And I had started to gain weight again. The 2016 election, depression, old habits... for the first time in years, my body felt unfamiliar.
Tweet! Tweet! We're back!
Nice to see you! Forget your running!
But I was determined. I would ignore my body, and be VICTORIOUS.
I decided that for my 50th birthday, I would run a back-to-back 5K and half marathon.
Rock 'N' Roll Half
34226
LAS VEGAS
in...
LAS VEGAS!

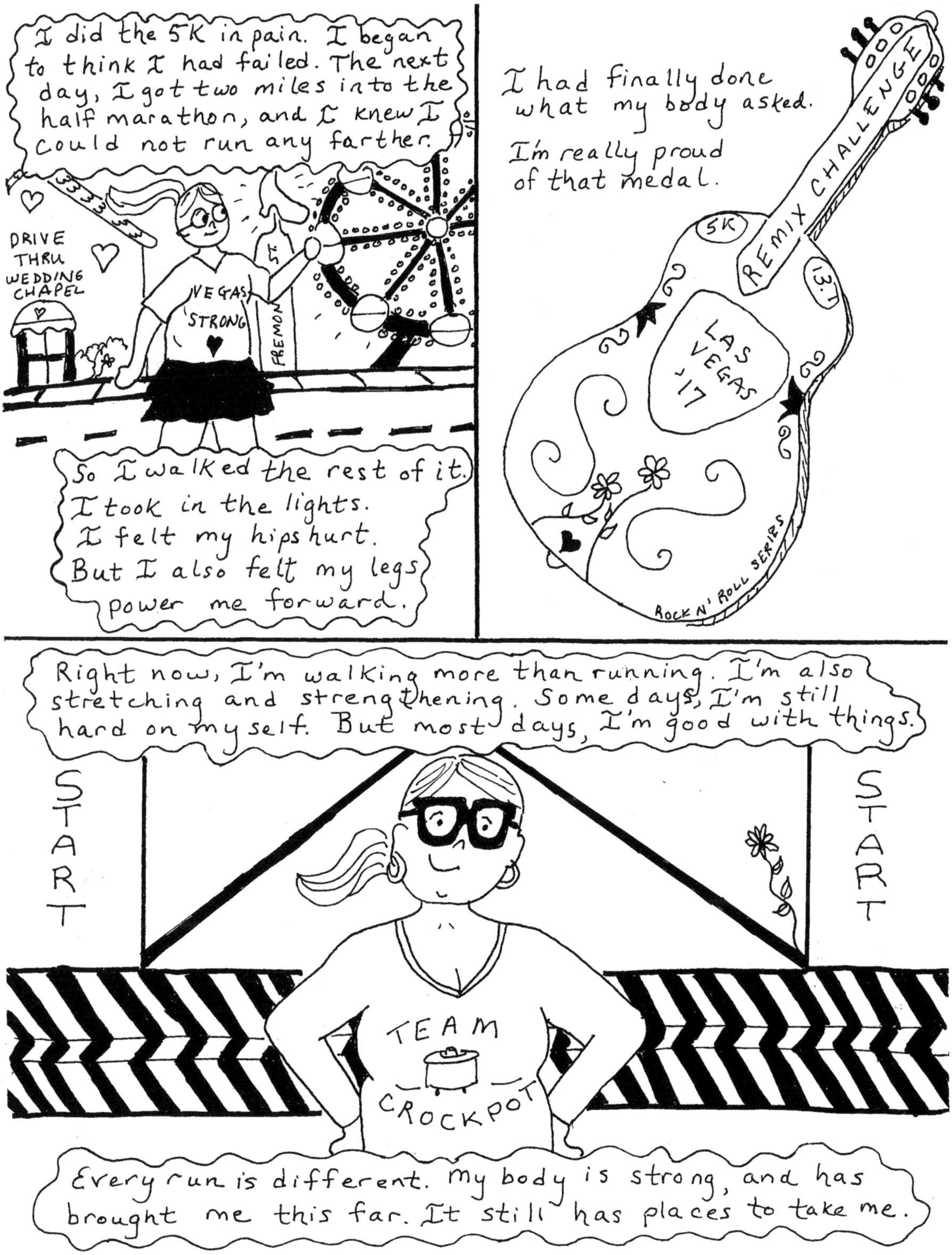
I did the 5K in pain. I began to think I had failed. The next day, I got two miles into the half marathon, and I knew I could not run any farther.
DRIVE THRU WEDDING CHAPEL
VEGAS STRONG
FREMONT ST.
So I walked the rest of it. I took in the lights. I felt my hips hurt. But I also felt my legs power me forward.
I had finally done what my body asked.
I'm really proud of that medal.
REMIX CHALLENGE
5K
13.1
LAS VEGAS '17
ROCK N' ROLL SERIES
Right now, I'm walking more than running. I'm also stretching and strengthening. Some days, I'm still hard on myself. But most days, I'm good with things.
START
START
TEAM CROCKPOT
Every run is different. My body is strong, and has brought me this far. It still has places to take me.

WHEN MY BIOLOGICAL CLOCK STOPPED TICKING

Here is the thing. If you ask me about menopause...

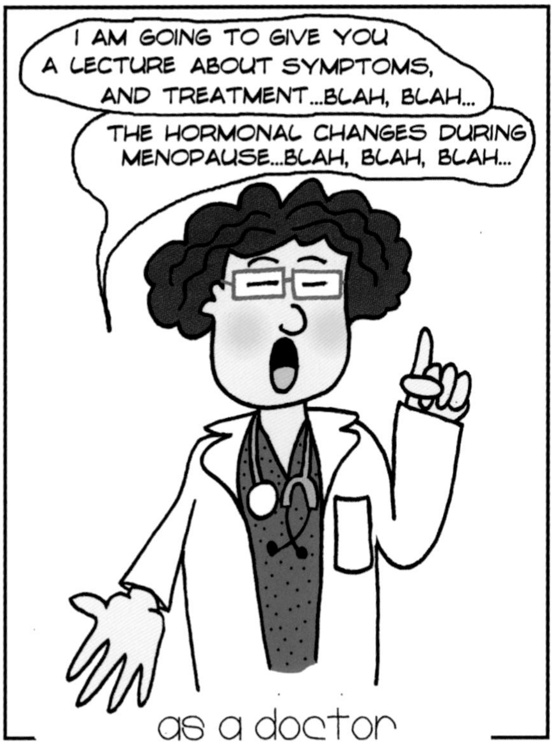
I AM GOING TO GIVE YOU A LECTURE ABOUT SYMPTOMS, AND TREATMENT...BLAH, BLAH...
THE HORMONAL CHANGES DURING MENOPAUSE...BLAH, BLAH, BLAH...
as a doctor

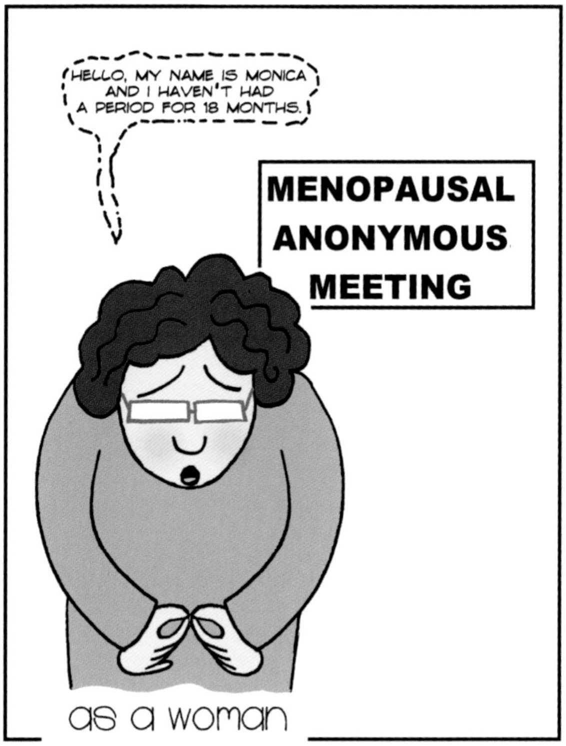
HELLO, MY NAME IS MONICA AND I HAVEN'T HAD A PERIOD FOR 18 MONTHS.
MENOPAUSAL ANONYMOUS MEETING
as a woman

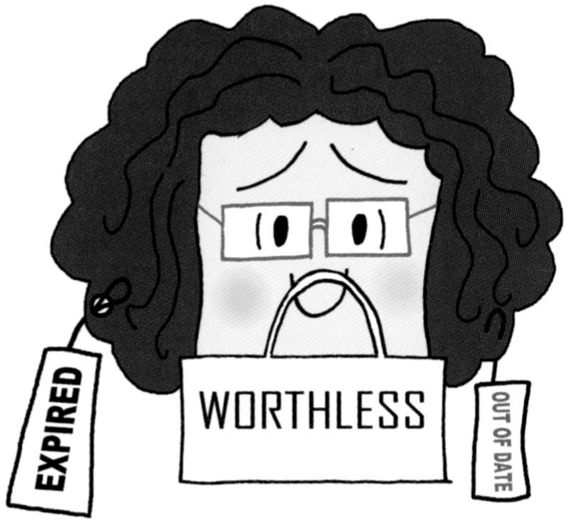
EXPIRED
WORTHLESS
OUT OF DATE

I can describe the feeling about my own menopause with one single word:
SHAME
But why?

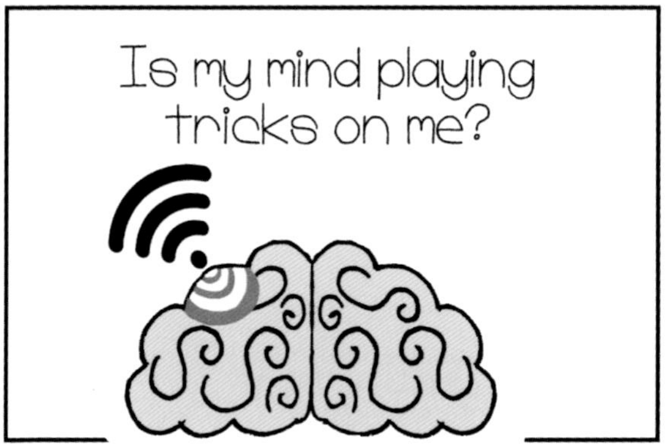
Is my mind playing tricks on me?

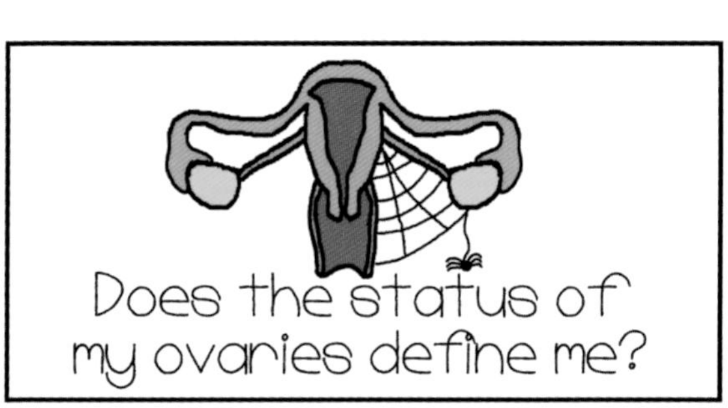
Does the status of my ovaries define me?

Women over 45 years old

We may sense life like this...

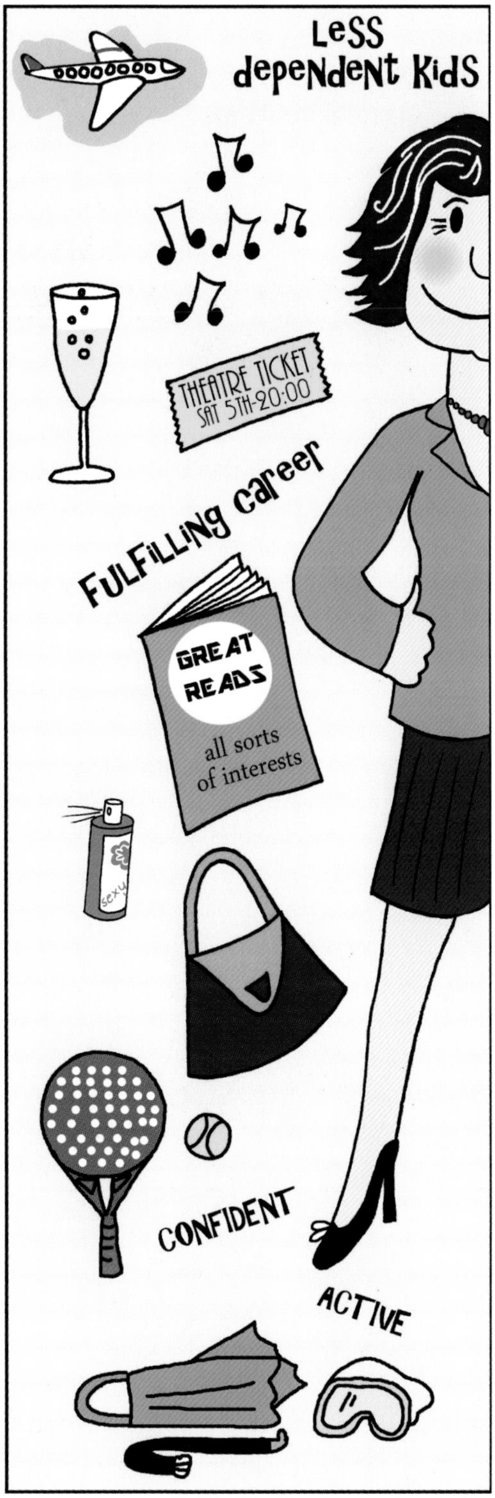
LeSS dependent KidS
THEATRE TICKET SAT 5TH-20:00
FULFILLING career
GREAT READS
all sorts of interests
sexy
CONFIDENT
ACTIVE

But we get bombarded like this...

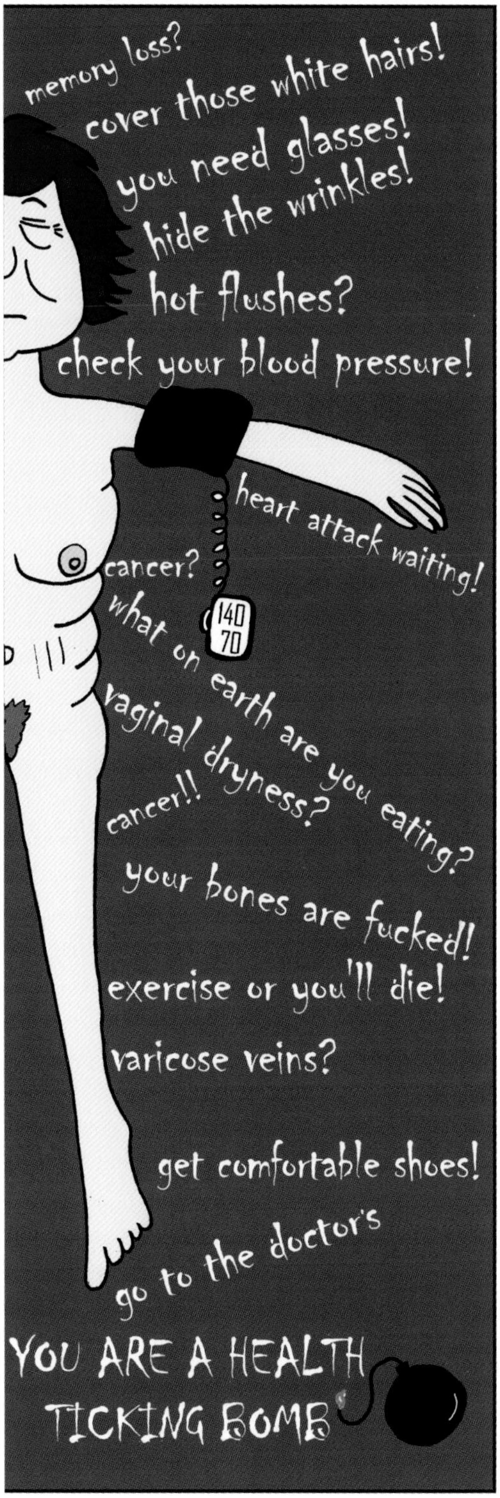
memory loss?
cover those white hairs!
you need glasses!
hide the wrinkles!
hot flushes?
check your blood pressure!
heart attack waiting!
cancer?
140
70
what on earth are you eating?
vaginal dryness?
cancer!!
your bones are fucked!
exercise or you'll die!
varicose veins?
get comfortable shoes!
go to the doctor's
YOU ARE A HEALTH TICKING BOMB

Pay attention to adverts with middle-aged women:

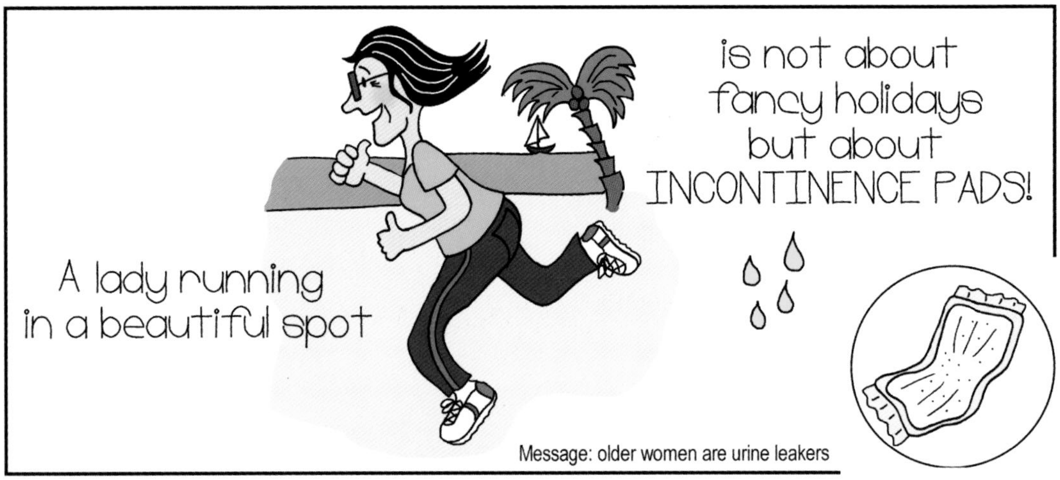
A lady running in a beautiful spot
is not about fancy holidays but about INCONTINENCE PADS!
Message: older women are urine leakers

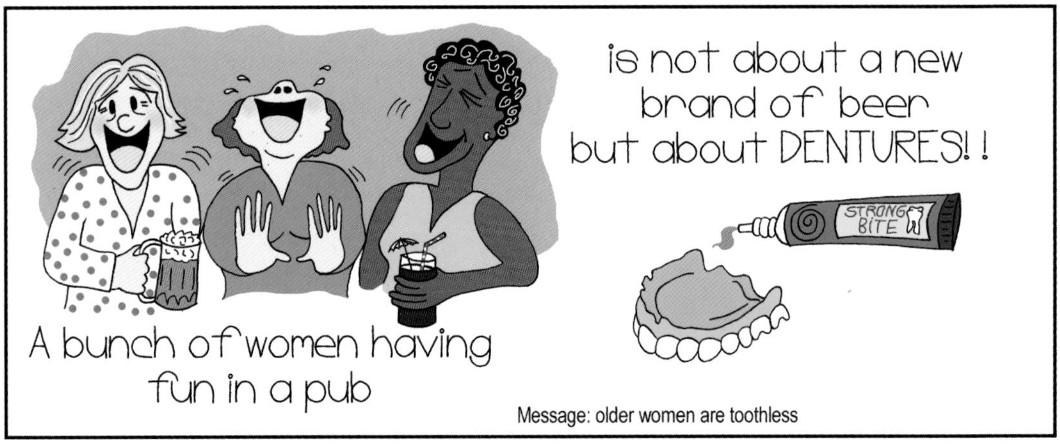
A bunch of women having fun in a pub
is not about a new brand of beer but about DENTURES! !
STRONG BITE
Message: older women are toothless

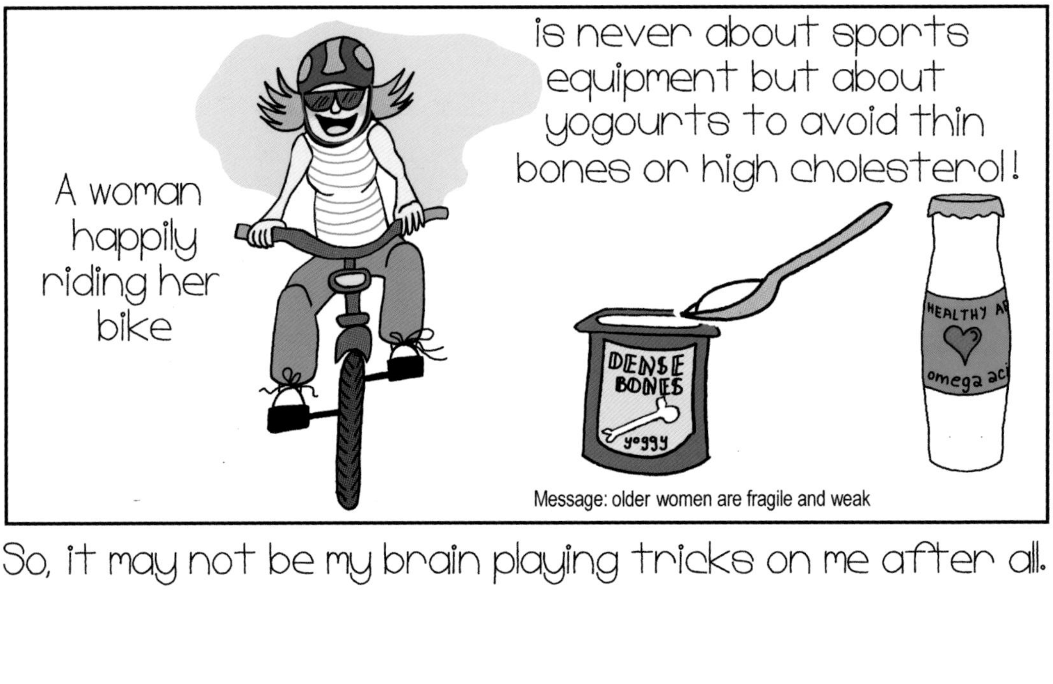
A woman happily riding her bike
is never about sports equipment but about yogourts to avoid thin bones or high cholesterol!
DENSE BONES
yoggy
HEALTHY A
omega ac
Message: older women are fragile and weak

So, it may not be my brain playing tricks on me after all.

My own Menopausal process

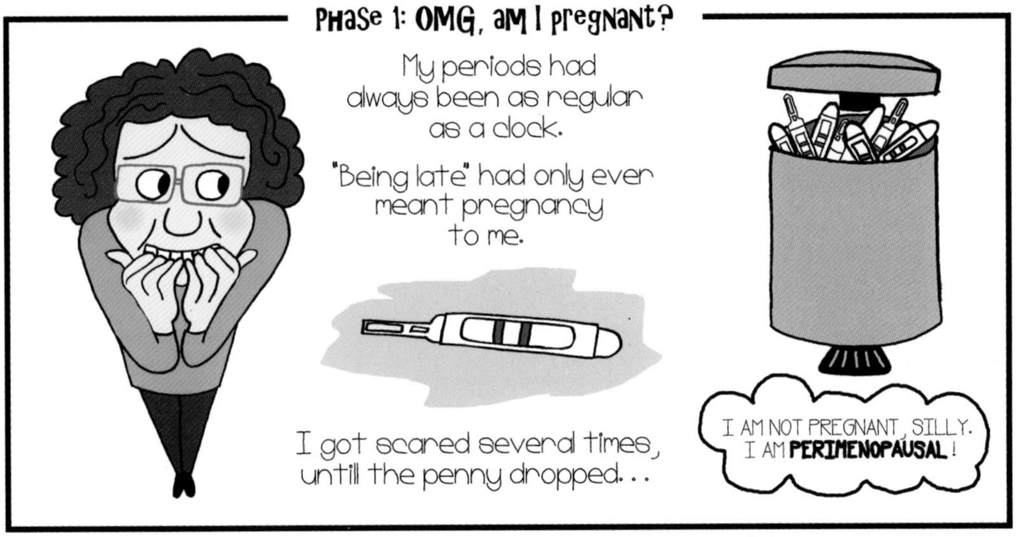
Phase 1: OMG, am I pregnant?
My periods had always been as regular as a clock.
"Being late" had only ever meant pregnancy to me.
I got scared several times, until the penny dropped...
I AM NOT PREGNANT, SILLY. I AM **PERIMENOPAUSAL**!

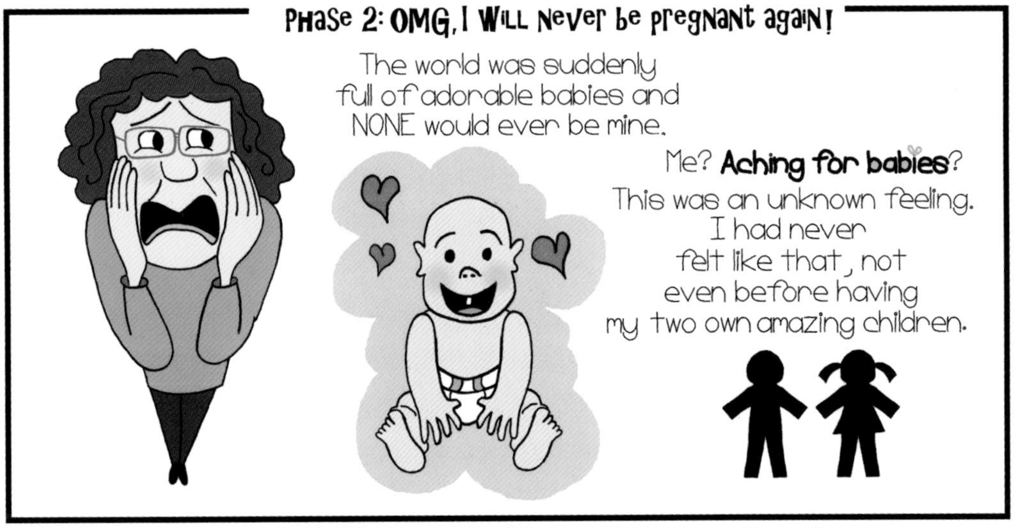
Phase 2: OMG, I will never be pregnant again!
The world was suddenly full of adorable babies and NONE would ever be mine.
Me? **Aching for babies**?
This was an unknown feeling. I had never felt like that, not even before having my two own amazing children.

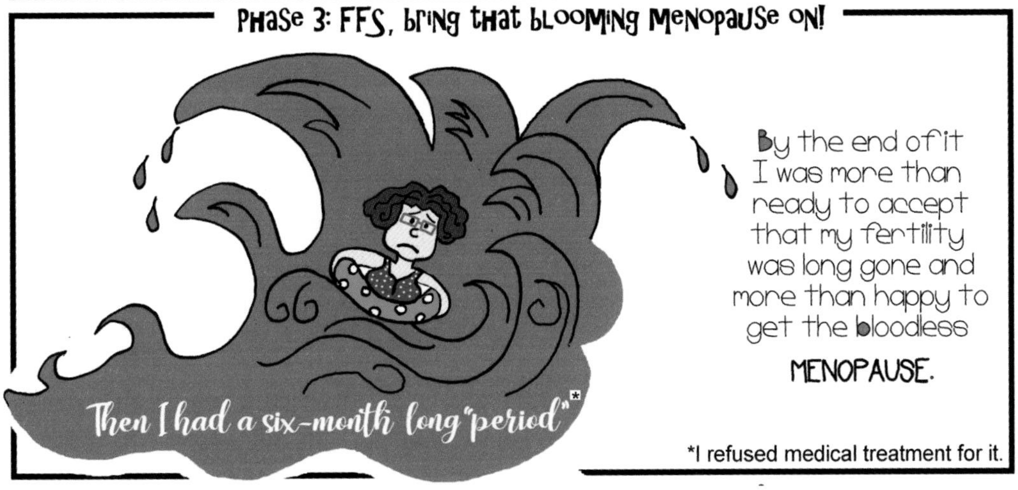
Phase 3: FFS, bring that blooming menopause on!
By the end of it I was more than ready to accept that my fertility was long gone and more than happy to get the bloodless
MENOPAUSE.
Then I had a six-month long "period"*
*I refused medical treatment for it.

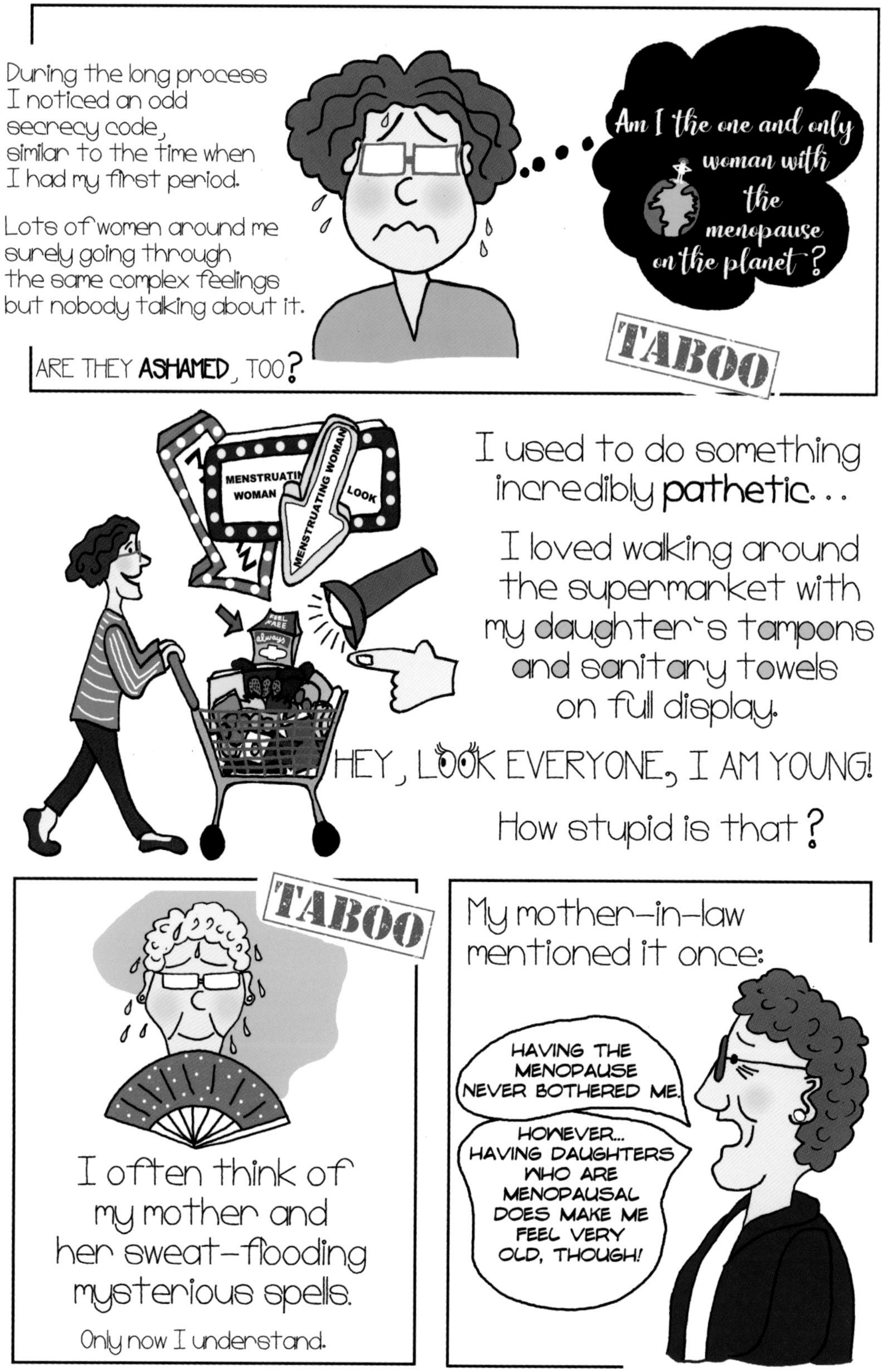
During the long process
I noticed an odd
secrecy code,
similar to the time when
I had my first period.
Lots of women around me
surely going through
the same complex feelings
but nobody talking about it.
Am I the one and only woman with the menopause on the planet?
ARE THEY **ASHAMED**, TOO?
TABOO
MENSTRUATING WOMAN
MENSTRUATING WOMAN
LOOK
FEEL FREE
always
I used to do something
incredibly **pathetic**...
I loved walking around
the supermarket with
my daughter's tampons
and sanitary towels
on full display.
HEY, LOOK EVERYONE, I AM YOUNG!
How stupid is that?
TABOO
I often think of
my mother and
her sweat-flooding
mysterious spells.
Only now I understand.
My mother-in-law
mentioned it once:
HAVING THE MENOPAUSE NEVER BOTHERED ME.
HOWEVER... HAVING DAUGHTERS WHO ARE MENOPAUSAL DOES MAKE ME FEEL VERY OLD, THOUGH!

Here is my message:

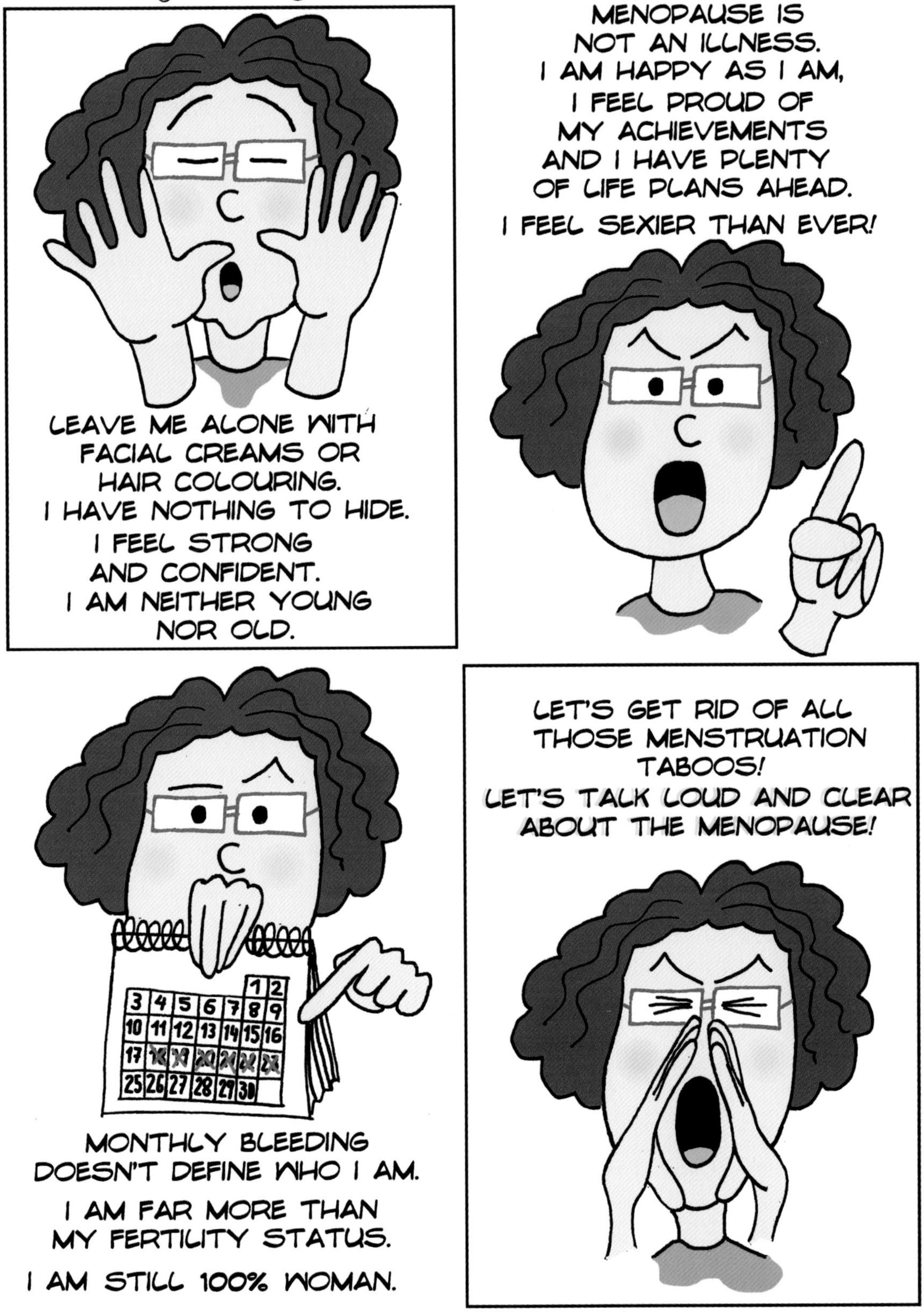
LEAVE ME ALONE WITH FACIAL CREAMS OR HAIR COLOURING.
I HAVE NOTHING TO HIDE.
I FEEL STRONG AND CONFIDENT.
I AM NEITHER YOUNG NOR OLD.
MENOPAUSE IS NOT AN ILLNESS.
I AM HAPPY AS I AM,
I FEEL PROUD OF MY ACHIEVEMENTS AND I HAVE PLENTY OF LIFE PLANS AHEAD.
I FEEL SEXIER THAN EVER!
MONTHLY BLEEDING DOESN'T DEFINE WHO I AM.
I AM FAR MORE THAN MY FERTILITY STATUS.
I AM STILL 100% WOMAN.
LET'S GET RID OF ALL THOSE MENSTRUATION TABOOS!
LET'S TALK LOUD AND CLEAR ABOUT THE MENOPAUSE!

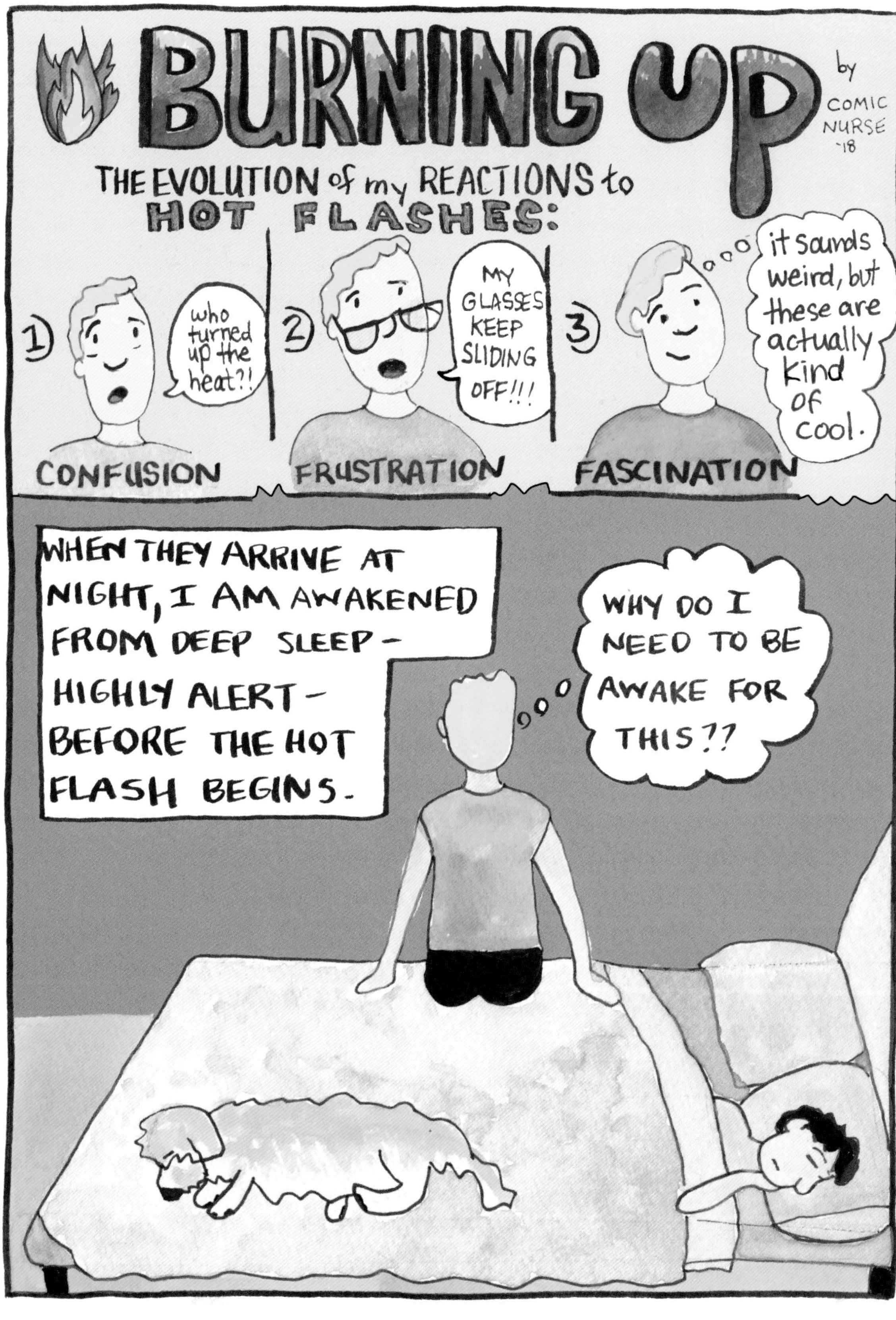

BURNING UP
by COMIC NURSE '18
THE EVOLUTION of my REACTIONS to HOT FLASHES:
1)
who turned up the heat?!
CONFUSION
2)
MY GLASSES KEEP SLIDING OFF!!!
FRUSTRATION
3)
it sounds weird, but these are actually kind of cool.
FASCINATION
WHEN THEY ARRIVE AT NIGHT, I AM AWAKENED FROM DEEP SLEEP - HIGHLY ALERT - BEFORE THE HOT FLASH BEGINS.
WHY DO I NEED TO BE AWAKE FOR THIS?!

Burning Up

32

Comic Nurse (MK Czerwiec)

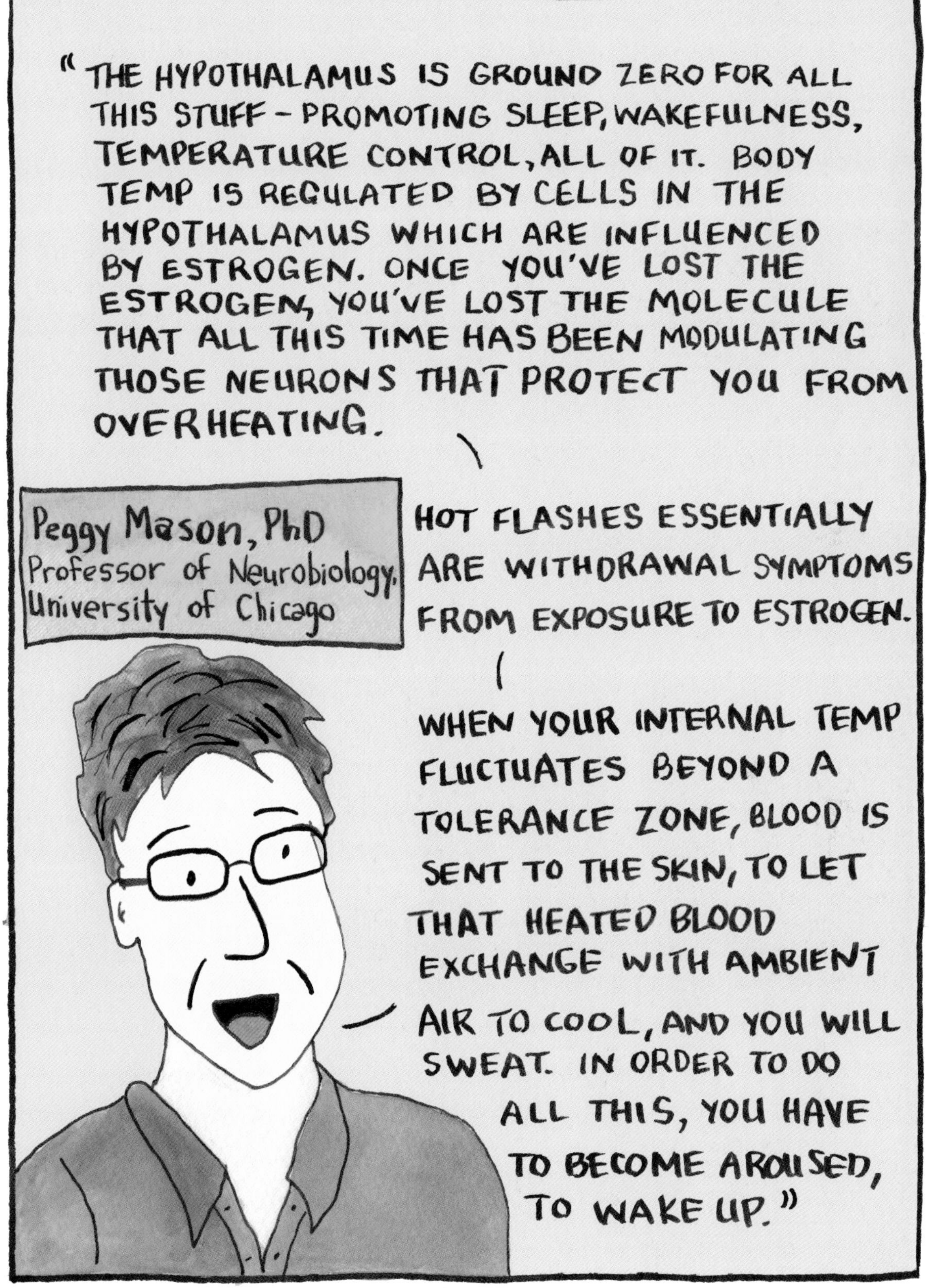

"THE HYPOTHALAMUS IS GROUND ZERO FOR ALL THIS STUFF — PROMOTING SLEEP, WAKEFULNESS, TEMPERATURE CONTROL, ALL OF IT. BODY TEMP IS REGULATED BY CELLS IN THE HYPOTHALAMUS WHICH ARE INFLUENCED BY ESTROGEN. ONCE YOU'VE LOST THE ESTROGEN, YOU'VE LOST THE MOLECULE THAT ALL THIS TIME HAS BEEN MODULATING THOSE NEURONS THAT PROTECT YOU FROM OVERHEATING.

Peggy Mason, PhD
Professor of Neurobiology, University of Chicago

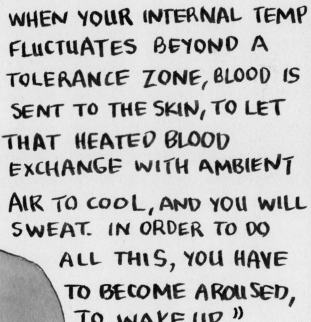

HOT FLASHES ESSENTIALLY ARE WITHDRAWAL SYMPTOMS FROM EXPOSURE TO ESTROGEN.

WHEN YOUR INTERNAL TEMP FLUCTUATES BEYOND A TOLERANCE ZONE, BLOOD IS SENT TO THE SKIN, TO LET THAT HEATED BLOOD EXCHANGE WITH AMBIENT AIR TO COOL, AND YOU WILL SWEAT. IN ORDER TO DO ALL THIS, YOU HAVE TO BECOME AROUSED, TO WAKE UP."

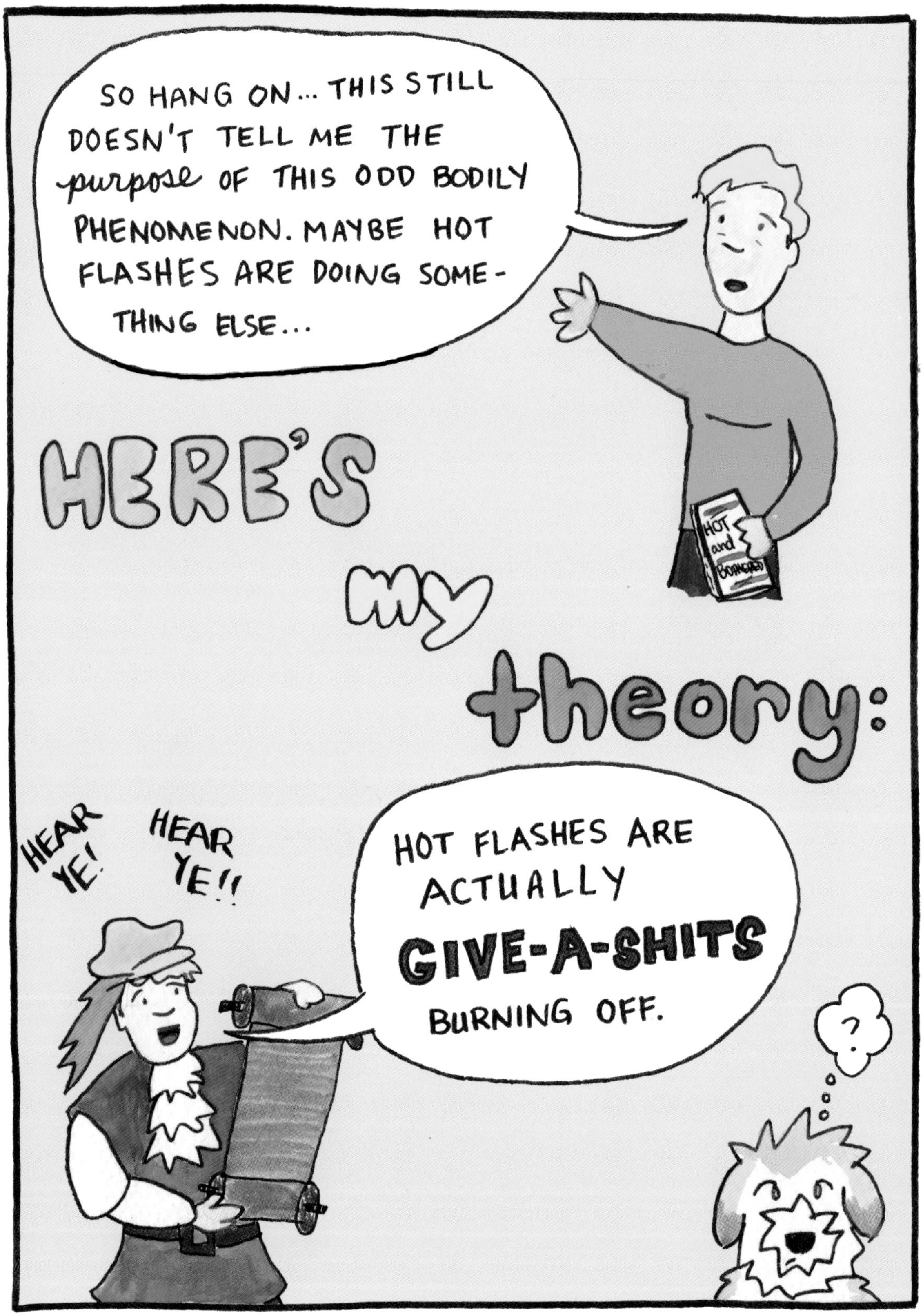
SO HANG ON... THIS STILL DOESN'T TELL ME THE *purpose* OF THIS ODD BODILY PHENOMENON. MAYBE HOT FLASHES ARE DOING SOME-THING ELSE...
HOT and BOTHERED
HERE'S my theory:
HEAR YE!
HEAR YE!!
HOT FLASHES ARE ACTUALLY **GIVE-A-SHITS** BURNING OFF.
?

POST-MENOPAUSAL WOMEN REPORT A SENSE OF FREEDOM NOT KNOWN IN YOUNGER YEARS.

I JUST DON'T GIVE A SHIT ANYMORE. I DON'T WORRY ABOUT ANY OF THE THINGS I WASTED TIME & ENERGY ON BEFORE.

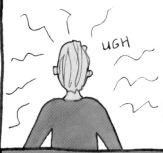

SO THAT'S WHAT HOT FLASHES ARE FOR, burning off all of our

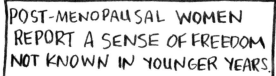

GIVE-A-SHITS!

WHAT PEOPLE THINK OF ME

UGH

NOT ASKING FOR HELP (when I need it)

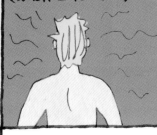

CHIN HAIRS

PHEW.

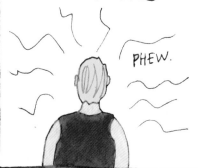

MY IMPERFECT BODY

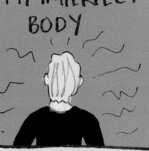

THAT THING I SAID BACK IN '92

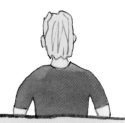

MY NEED FOR APPROVAL

SIGH.

(THIS ONE MAY TAKE A WHILE)

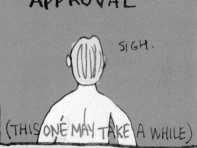

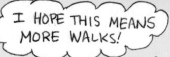

AND I NEED TO BE AWAKE TO NOTICE.

REALIZING THIS MADE ME RIDICULOUSLY HAPPY!!!

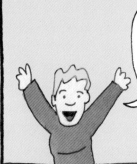

I HOPE THIS MEANS MORE WALKS!

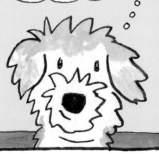

DESERTIFICATION

BY A.K. SUMMERS

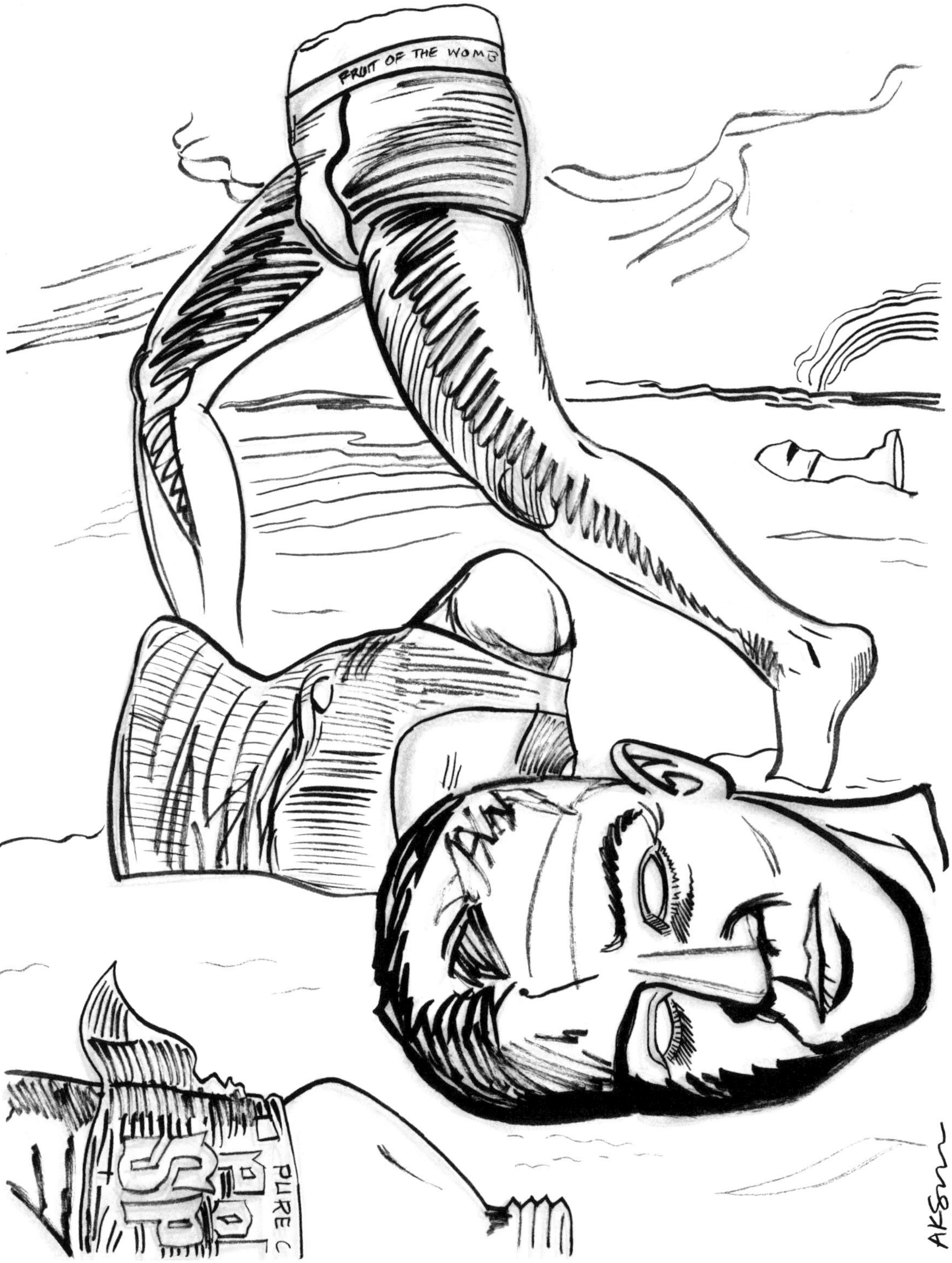
FRUIT OF THE WOMB

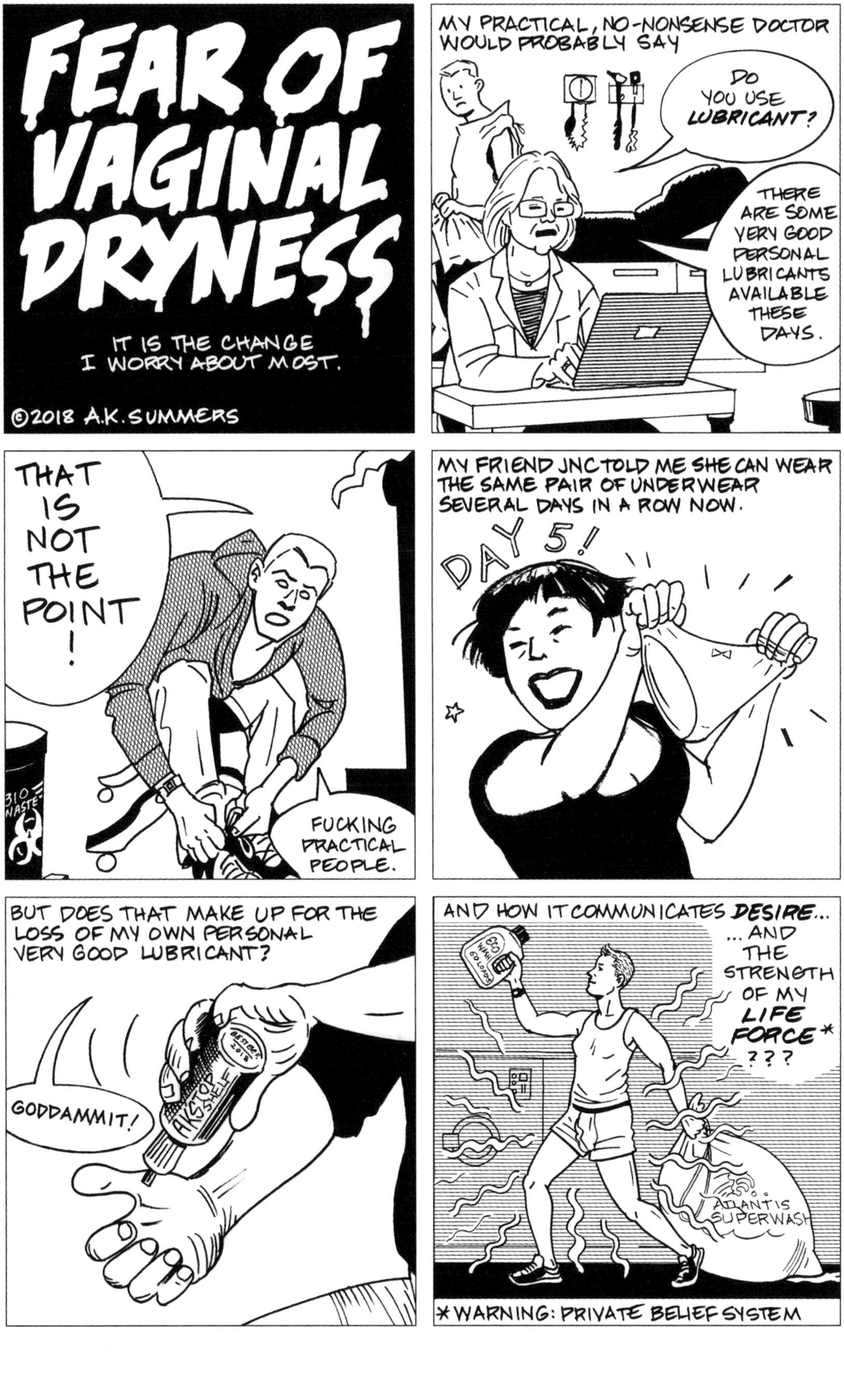
FEAR OF VAGINAL DRYNESS
IT IS THE CHANGE I WORRY ABOUT MOST.
©2018 A.K. SUMMERS
MY PRACTICAL, NO-NONSENSE DOCTOR WOULD PROBABLY SAY
DO YOU USE LUBRICANT?
THERE ARE SOME VERY GOOD PERSONAL LUBRICANTS AVAILABLE THESE DAYS.
THAT IS NOT THE POINT!
FUCKING PRACTICAL PEOPLE.
MY FRIEND JNC TOLD ME SHE CAN WEAR THE SAME PAIR OF UNDERWEAR SEVERAL DAYS IN A ROW NOW.
DAY 5!
BUT DOES THAT MAKE UP FOR THE LOSS OF MY OWN PERSONAL VERY GOOD LUBRICANT?
GODDAMMIT!
AND HOW IT COMMUNICATES DESIRE...
... AND THE STRENGTH OF MY LIFE FORCE* ???
ATLANTIS SUPERWASH
*WARNING: PRIVATE BELIEF SYSTEM

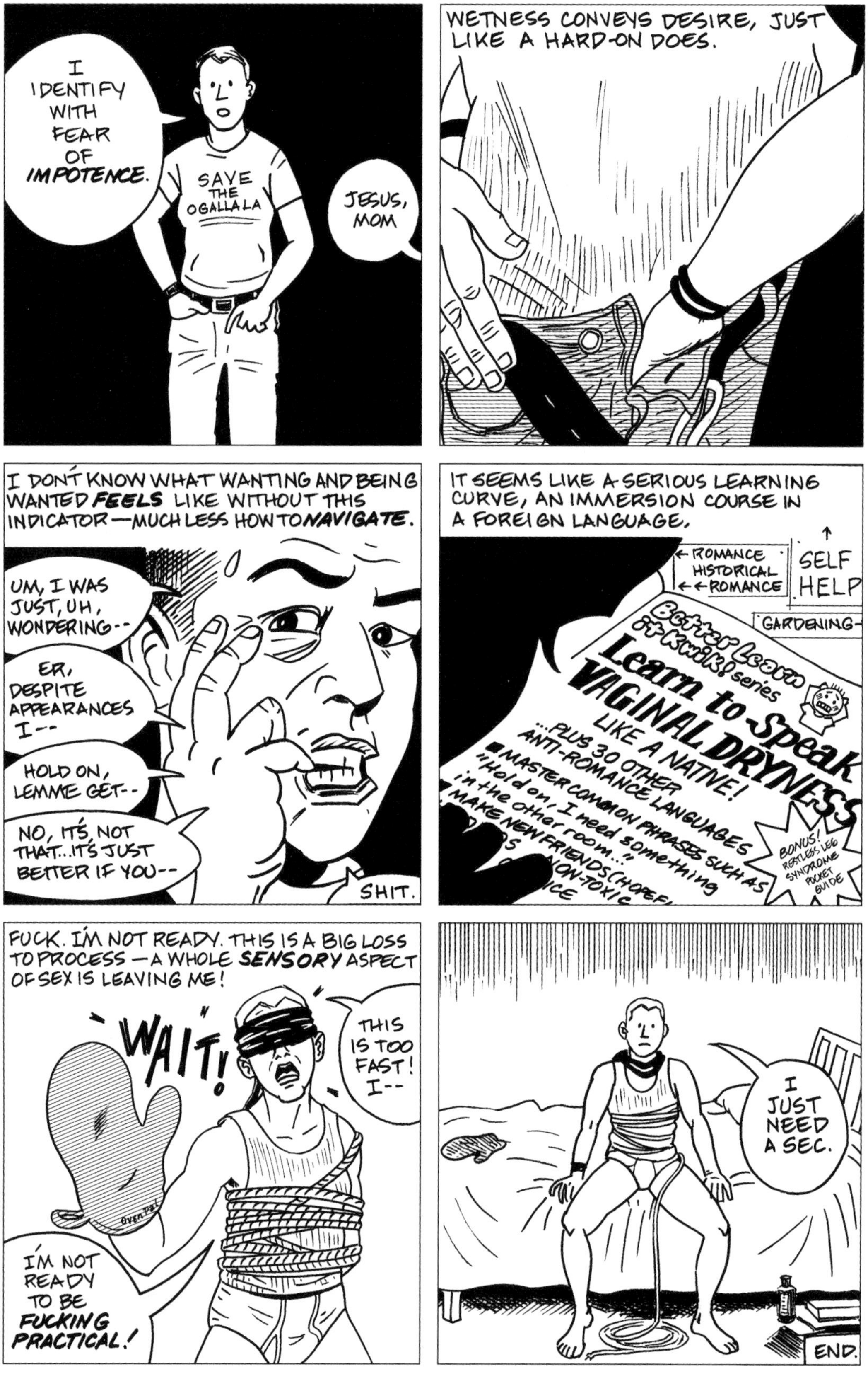
I IDENTIFY WITH FEAR OF *IMPOTENCE*.
SAVE THE OGALLALA
JESUS, MOM
WETNESS CONVEYS DESIRE, JUST LIKE A HARD-ON DOES.
I DON'T KNOW WHAT WANTING AND BEING WANTED **FEELS** LIKE WITHOUT THIS INDICATOR—MUCH LESS HOW TO **NAVIGATE**.
UM, I WAS JUST, UH, WONDERING--
ER, DESPITE APPEARANCES I--
HOLD ON, LEMME GET--
NO, IT'S NOT THAT...IT'S JUST BETTER IF YOU--
SHIT.
IT SEEMS LIKE A SERIOUS LEARNING CURVE, AN IMMERSION COURSE IN A FOREIGN LANGUAGE.
← ROMANCE
HISTORICAL ← ROMANCE
SELF HELP
GARDENING
Better Learn it Kwik! series
Learn to Speak VAGINAL DRYNESS LIKE A NATIVE!
...PLUS 30 OTHER ANTI-ROMANCE LANGUAGES
■ MASTER COMMON PHRASES SUCH AS "Hold on, I need something in the other room..."
■ MAKE NEW FRIENDS
BONUS! RESTLESS LEG SYNDROME POCKET GUIDE
FUCK. I'M NOT READY. THIS IS A BIG LOSS TO PROCESS—A WHOLE **SENSORY** ASPECT OF SEX IS LEAVING ME!
WAIT!
THIS IS TOO FAST! I--
I'M NOT READY TO BE **FUCKING PRACTICAL**!
I JUST NEED A SEC.
END.

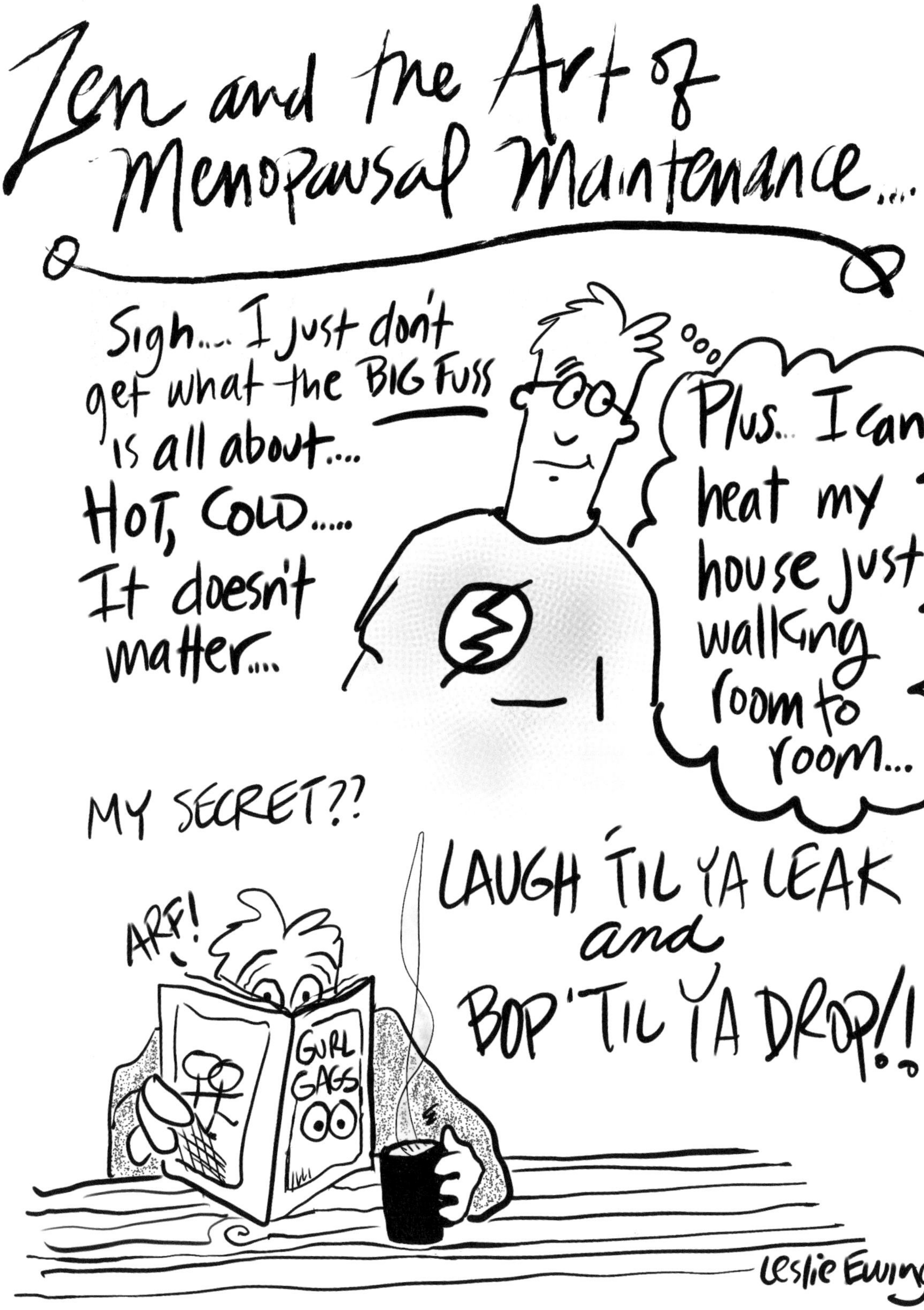
Zen and the Art of Menopausal Maintenance....
Sigh.... I just don't get what the BIG FUSS is all about.... HOT, COLD..... It doesn't matter....
Plus.. I can heat my house just walking room to room...
MY SECRET??
ARF!
GURL GASS
LAUGH 'TIL YA LEAK and BOP 'TIL YA DROP!!
Leslie Ewing

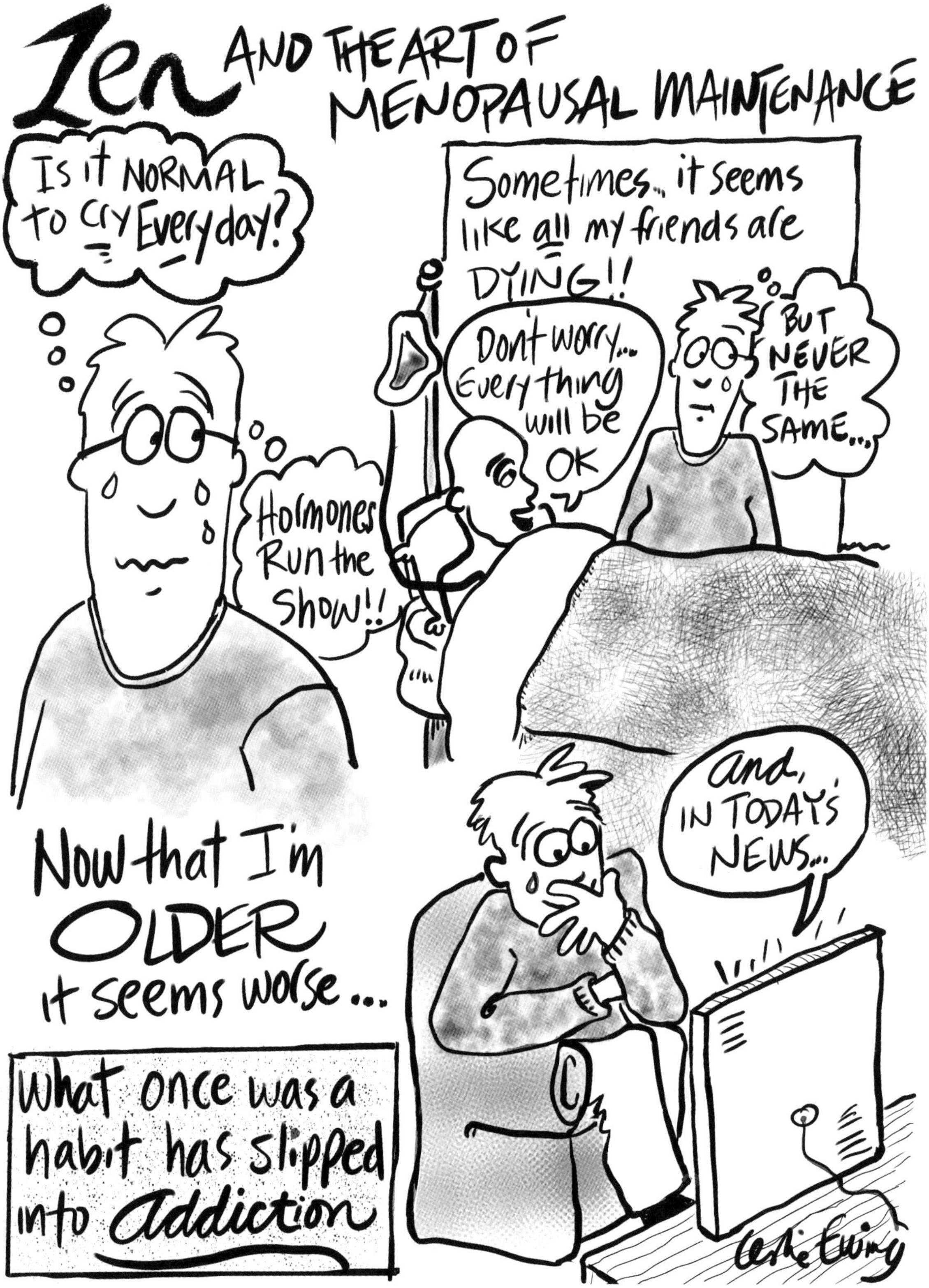
Zen AND THE ART OF MENOPAUSAL MAINTENANCE
Is it NORMAL to cry Everyday?
Hormones Run the Show!!
Sometimes... it seems like all my friends are DYING!!
Don't worry... Everything will be OK
BUT NEVER THE SAME...
Now that I'm OLDER it seems worse...
and, IN TODAY'S NEWS...
What once was a habit has slipped into addiction
Leslie Ewing

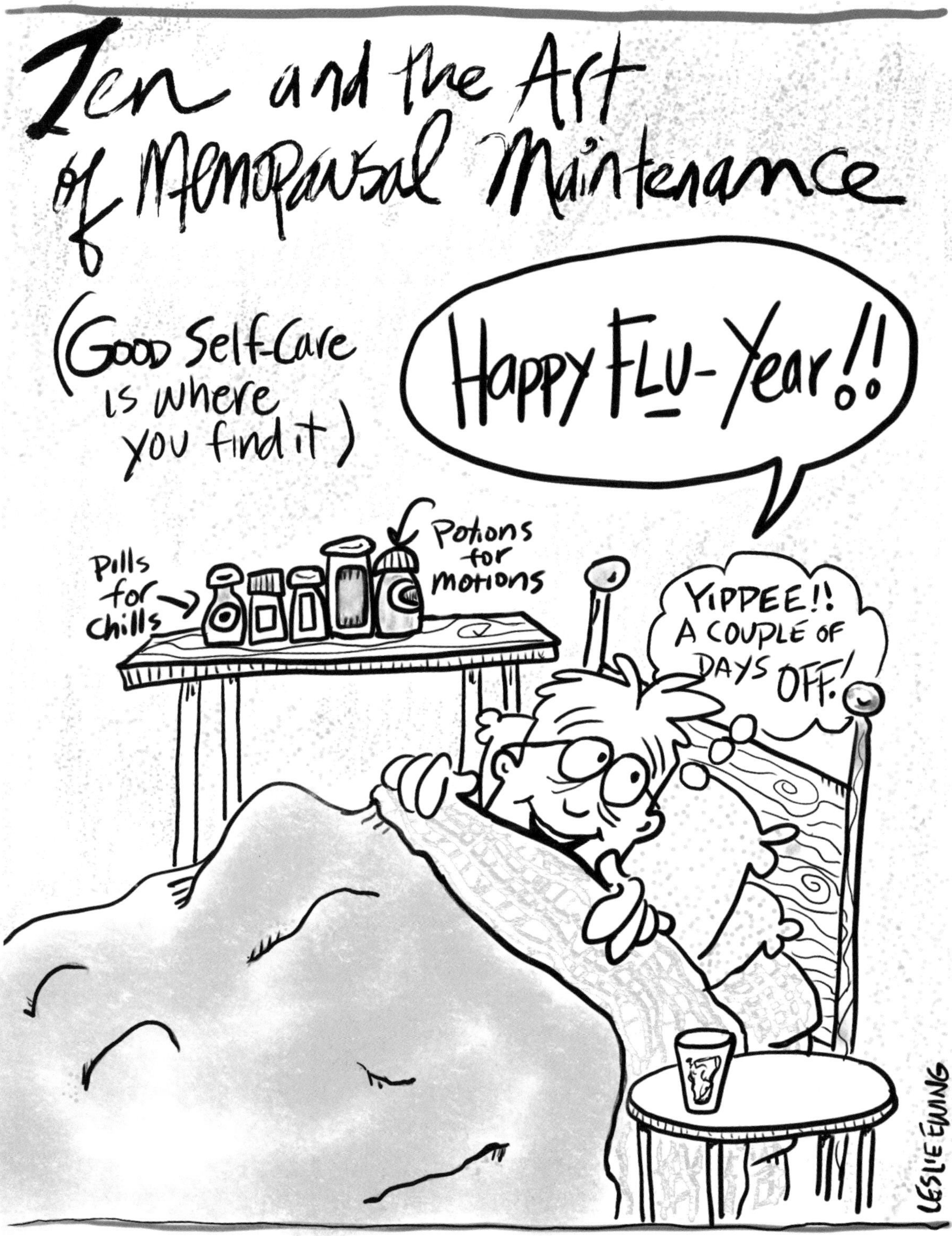
Zen and the Art of Menopausal Maintenance
(Good Self-Care is where you find it)
Happy FLU-Year!!
Pills for chills
Potions for motions
YIPPEE!! A COUPLE OF DAYS OFF!
LESLIE EWING

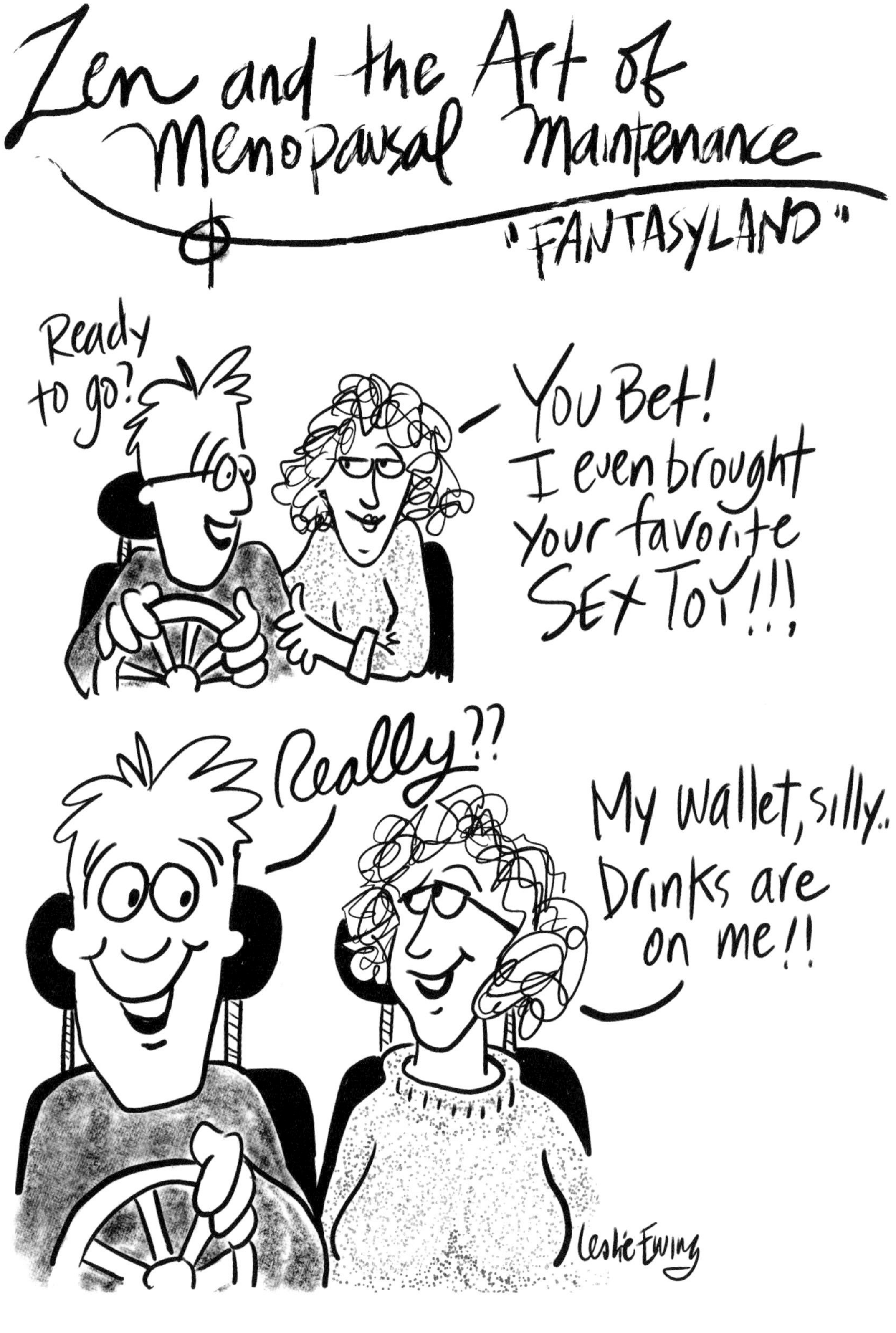
Zen and the Art of Menopausal Maintenance
"FANTASYLAND"
Ready to go?
You Bet! I even brought your favorite SEX TOY!!!
Really??
My wallet, silly.. Drinks are on me!!
Leslie Ewing

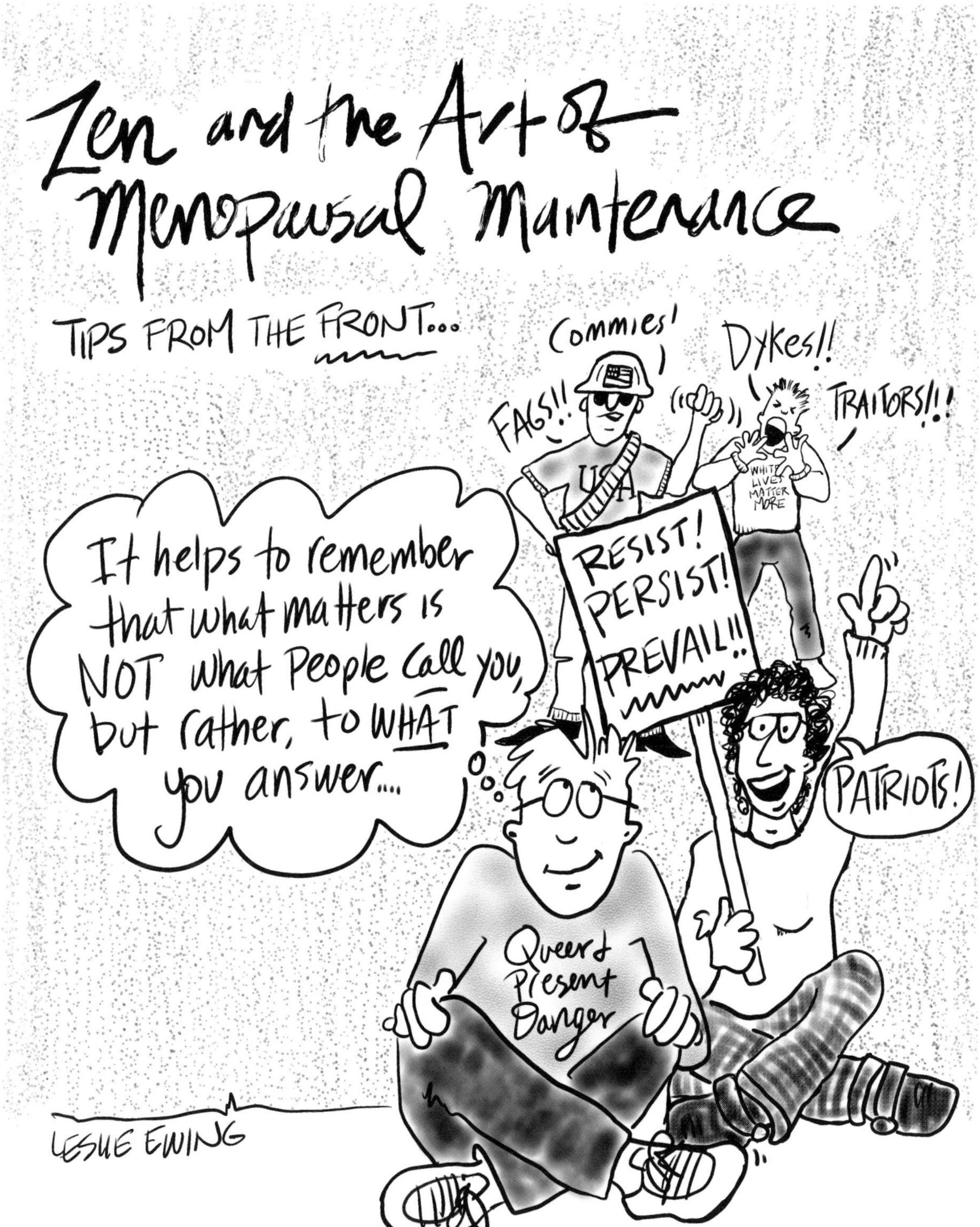
Zen and the Art of Menopausal Maintenance
TIPS FROM THE FRONT...
Commies!
Dykes!!
FAGS!!
TRAITORS!!!
USA
WHITE LIVES MATTER MORE
RESIST! PERSIST! PREVAIL!!
It helps to remember that what matters is NOT what People call you, but rather, to WHAT you answer....
PATRIOTS!
Queer & Present Danger
LESLIE EWING

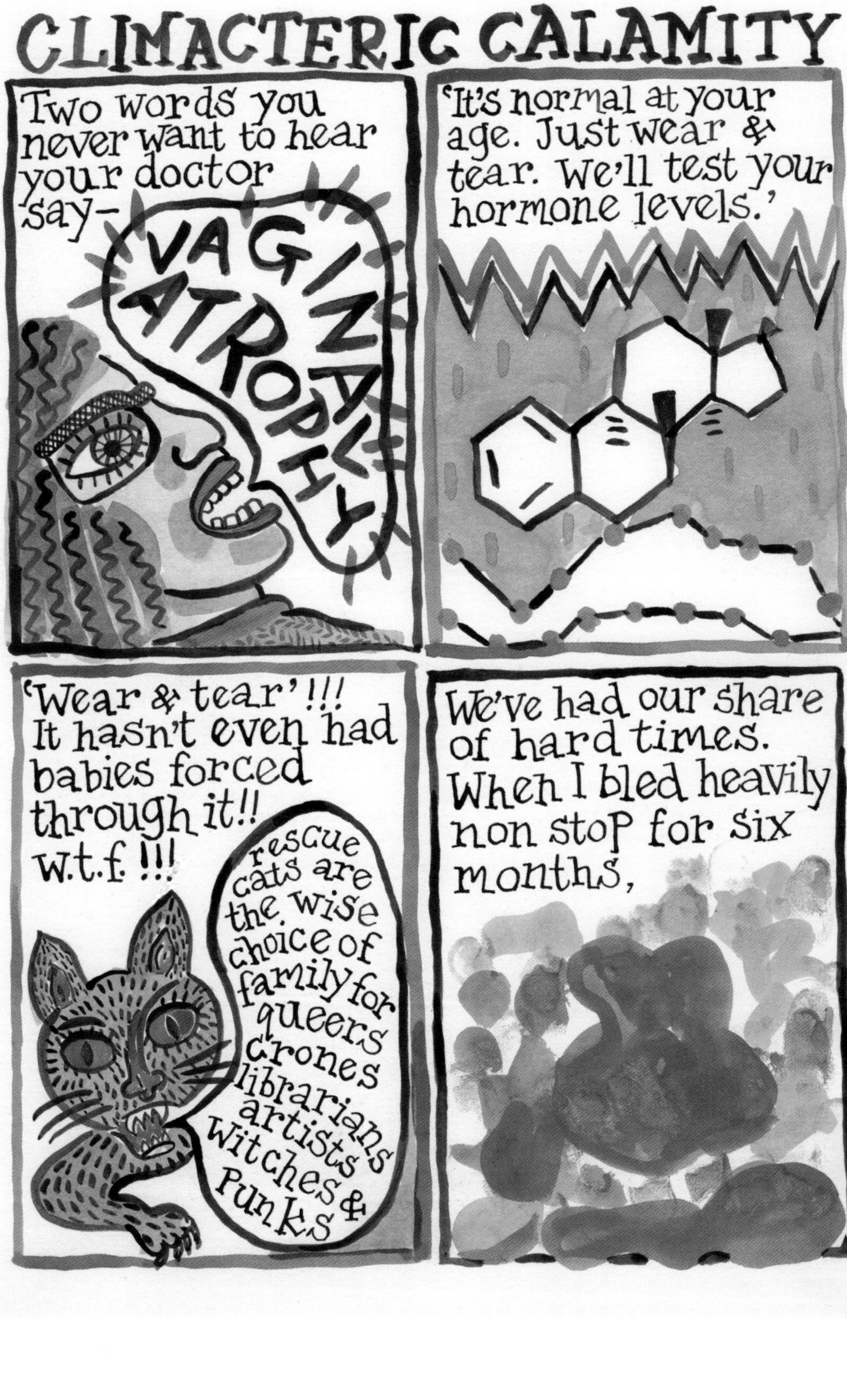

CLIMACTERIC CALAMITY

Two words you never want to hear your doctor say—

VAGINA ATROPHY

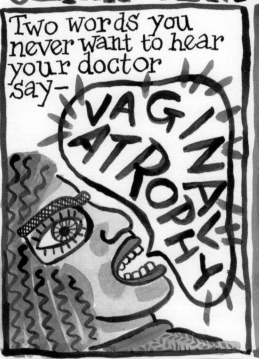

'It's normal at your age. Just wear & tear. We'll test your hormone levels.'

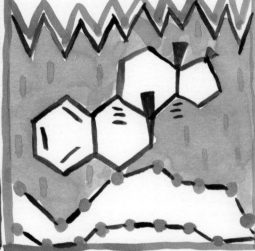

'Wear & tear'!!! It hasn't even had babies forced through it!! w.t.f.!!!

rescue cats are the wise choice of family for queers crones librarians artists witches & punks

We've had our share of hard times. When I bled heavily non stop for six months,

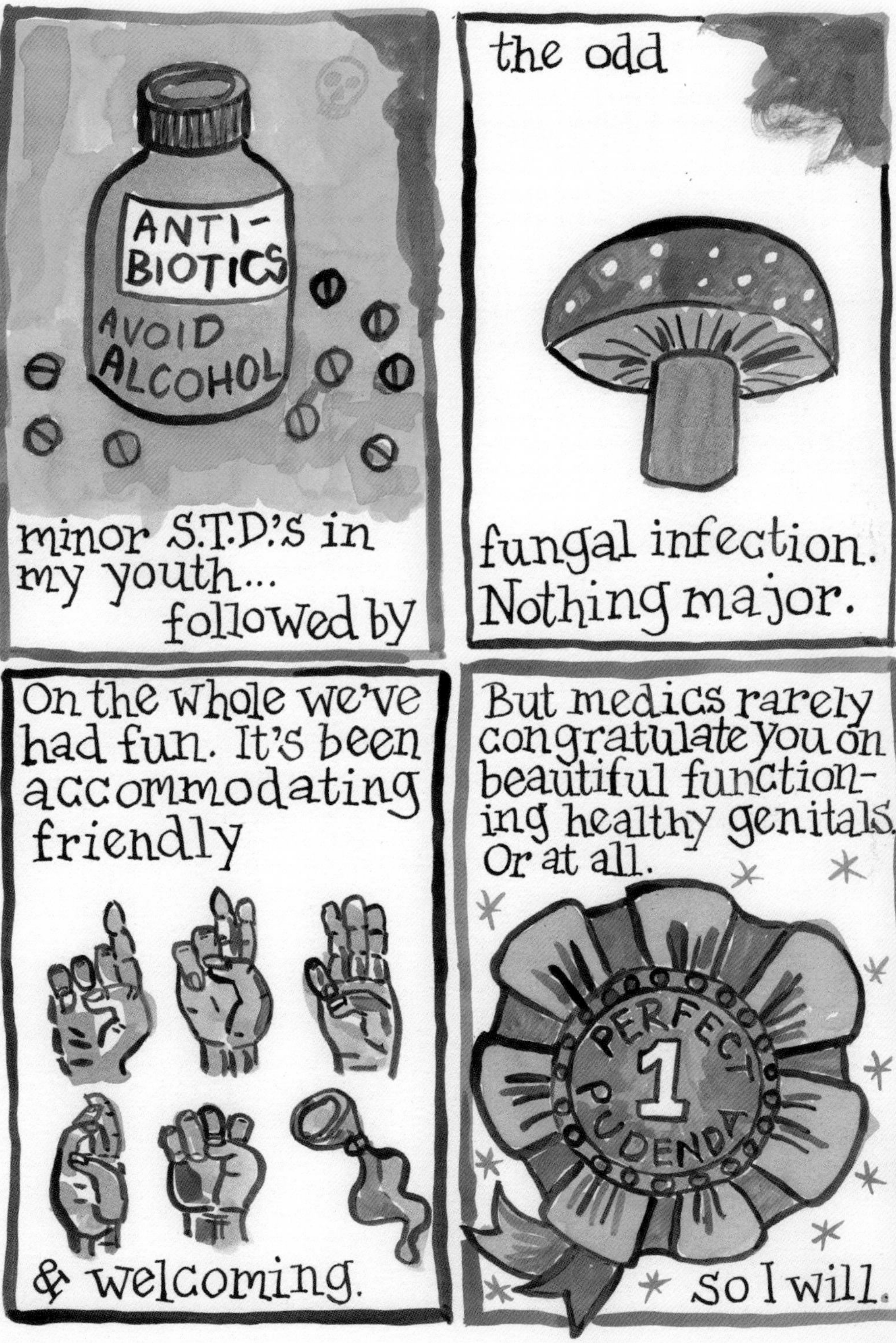

ANTI-BIOTICS
AVOID ALCOHOL
minor S.T.D.'s in my youth... followed by
the odd
fungal infection. Nothing major.
On the whole we've had fun. It's been accommodating friendly
& welcoming.
But medics rarely congratulate you on beautiful functioning healthy genitals. Or at all.
PERFECT 1 PUDENDA
so I will.

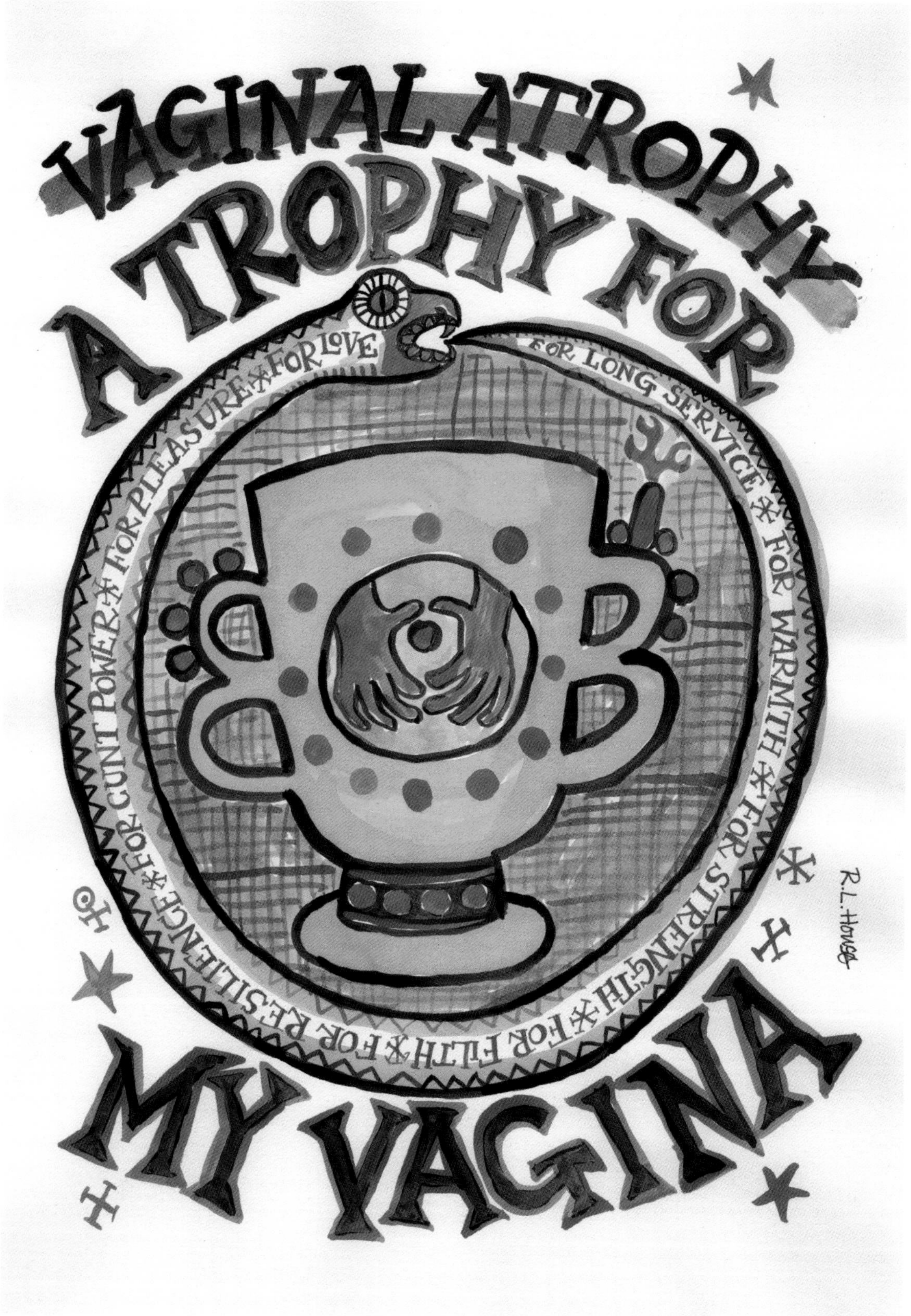
VAGINAL ATROPHY
A TROPHY FOR
FOR LOVE
FOR PLEASURE * FOR CUNT POWER * FOR RESILIENCE * FOR FILTH * FOR STRENGTH * FOR WARMTH * FOR LONG SERVICE
MY VAGINA
R.L. House

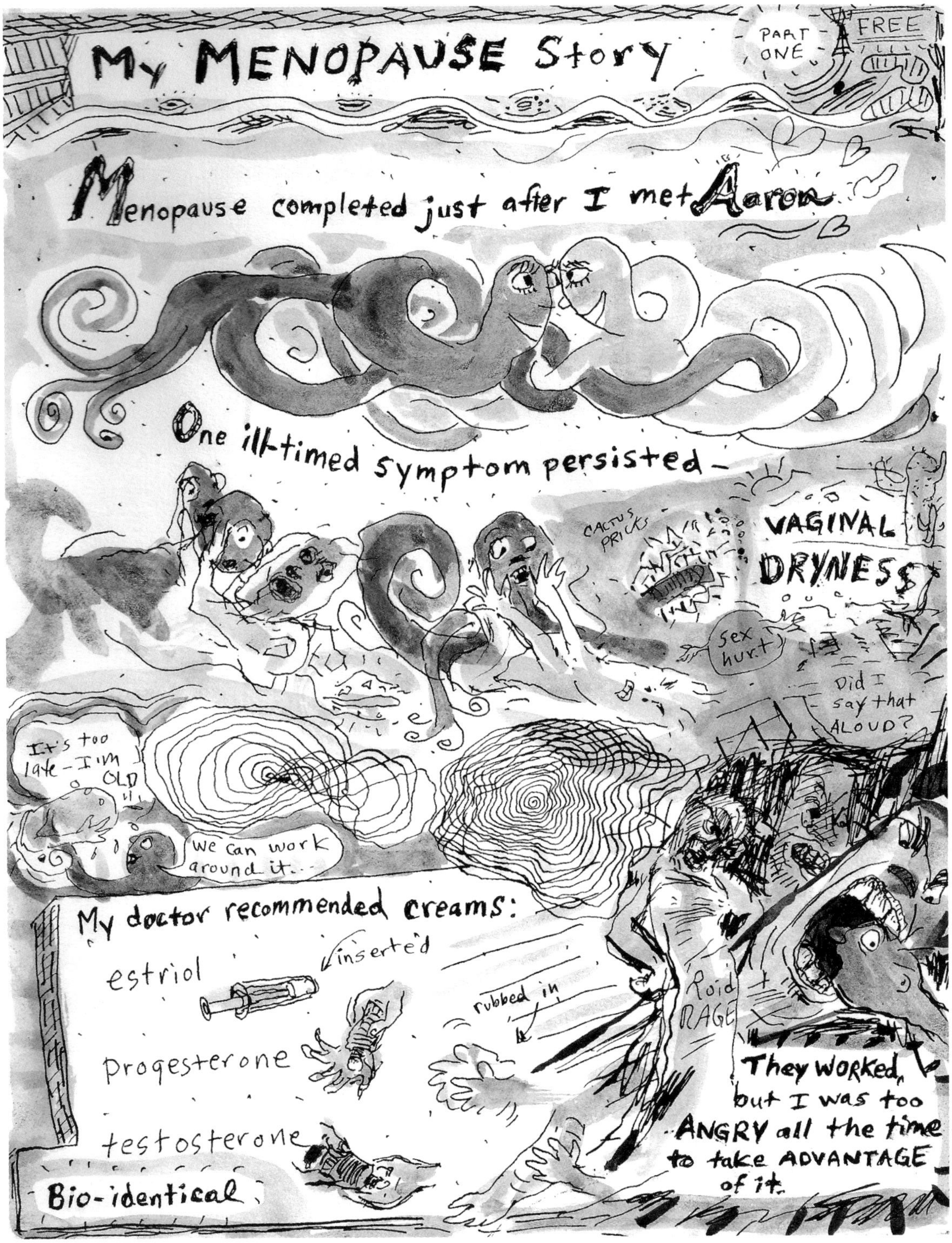

My MENOPAUSE Story
PART ONE
FREE
Menopause completed just after I met Aaron
One ill-timed symptom persisted –
CACTUS PRICKS
VAGINAL DRYNESS
Sex hurt
Did I say that ALOUD?
It's too late – I'm OLD
We can work around it.
My doctor recommended creams:
estriol
inserted
progesterone
rubbed in
testosterone
Bio-identical
Roid RAGE
They WORKED, but I was too ANGRY all the time to take ADVANTAGE of it.

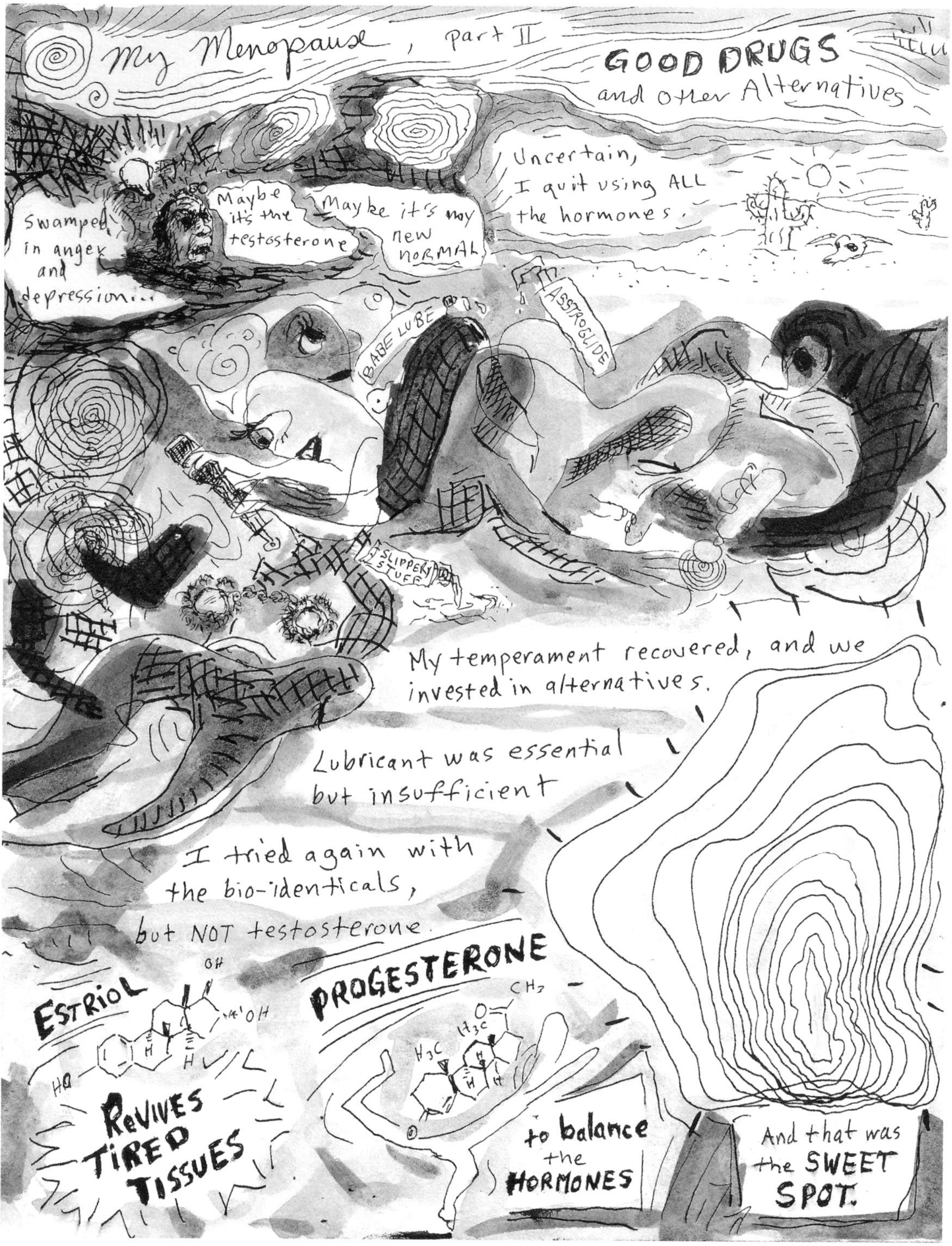

My Menopause, part II
GOOD DRUGS
and Other Alternatives
Swamped in anger and depression...
Maybe it's the testosterone
Maybe it's my new NORMAL
Uncertain, I quit using ALL the hormones.
BABE LUBE
ASTROGLIDE
SLIPPERY STUFF
My temperament recovered, and we invested in alternatives.
Lubricant was essential but insufficient
I tried again with the bio-identicals,
but NOT testosterone.
ESTRIOL
REVIVES TIRED TISSUES
PROGESTERONE
to balance the HORMONES
And that was the SWEET SPOT.

At the visit to your Urogynecologist you may be asked questions such as... "Are you sexually active?"

Well,
I'm Married...
Well...
he is.
Not Anymore!
Freedom 70!
Not Here.
This is "No Man's Land"

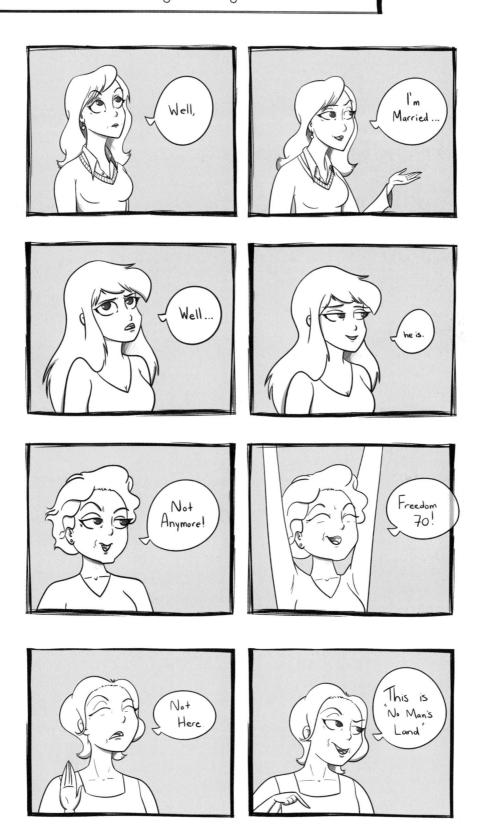

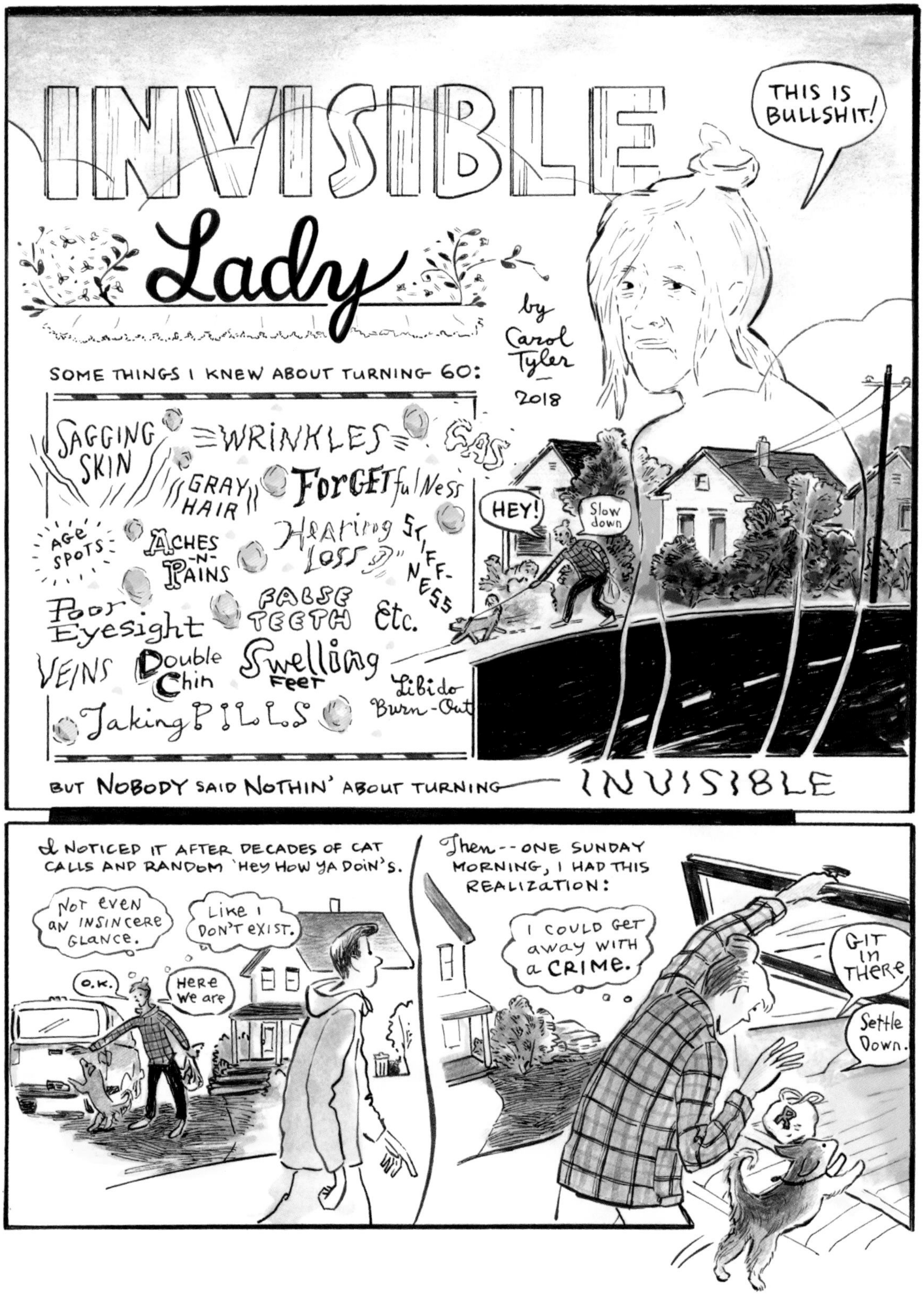
INVISIBLE
Lady
by Carol Tyler 2018
THIS IS BULLSHIT!
SOME THINGS I KNEW ABOUT TURNING 60:
SAGGING SKIN
WRINKLES
GAS
GRAY HAIR
FORGETfulNess
AGE SPOTS
ACHES -N- PAINS
Hearing LOSS
STIFF-NESS
Poor Eyesight
FALSE TEETH
Etc.
VEINS
Double Chin
Swelling FEET
Libido Burn-Out
Taking PILLS
HEY!
Slow down
BUT NOBODY SAID NOTHIN' ABOUT TURNING INVISIBLE
I NOTICED IT AFTER DECADES OF CAT CALLS AND RANDOM 'HEY HOW YA DOIN'S.
Not even an INSINCERE GLANCE.
Like I DON'T EXIST.
O.K.
Here we are
Then-- ONE SUNDAY MORNING, I HAD THIS REALIZATION:
I COULD GET away WITH a CRIME.
GIT IN THERE
Settle Down.

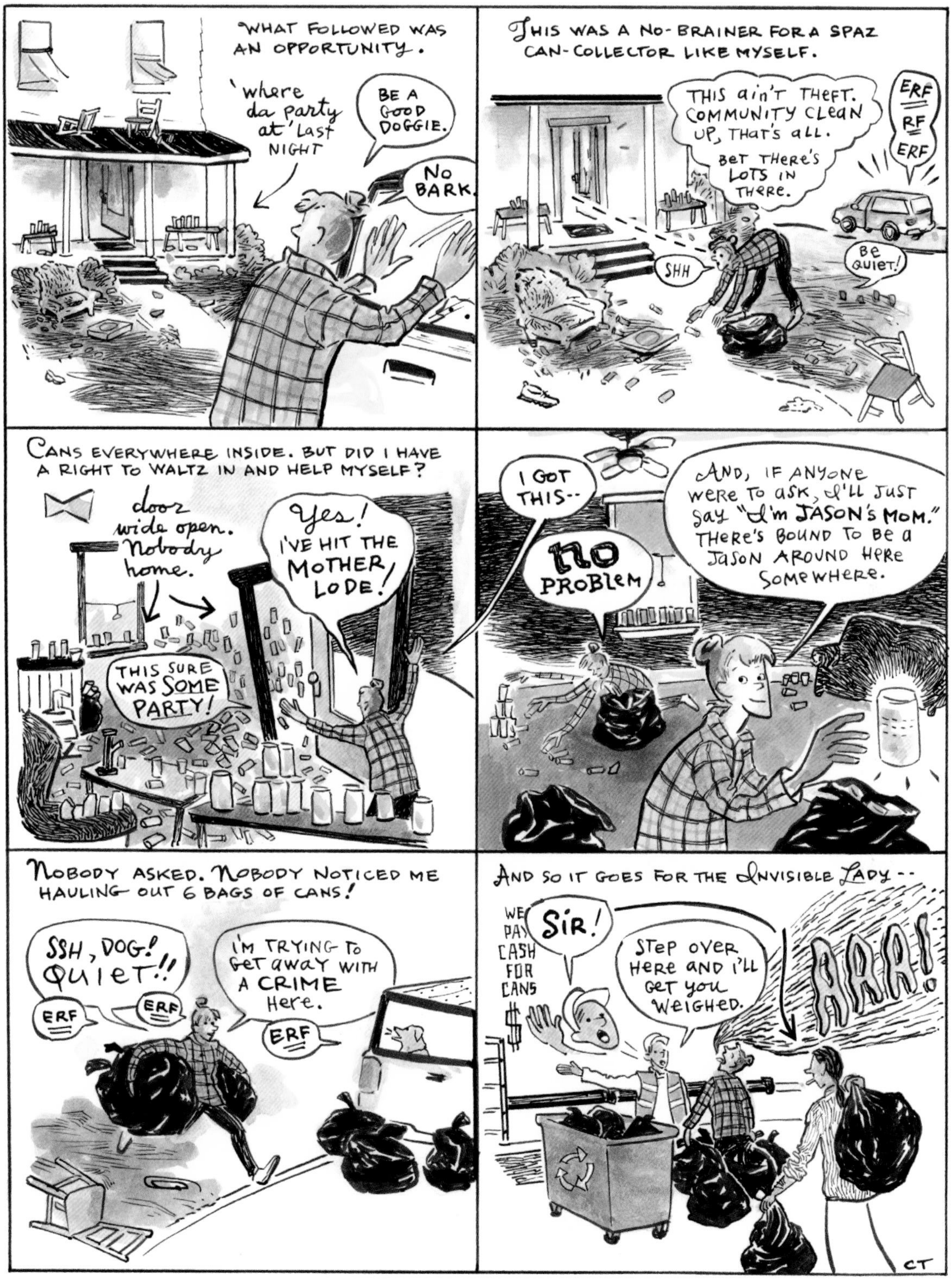
WHAT FOLLOWED WAS AN OPPORTUNITY.
where da party at last NIGHT
BE A GOOD DOGGIE.
NO BARK.
THIS WAS A NO-BRAINER FOR A SPAZ CAN-COLLECTOR LIKE MYSELF.
THIS ain't THEFT. COMMUNITY CLEAN UP, THAT'S ALL.
BET THERE'S LOTS IN THERE.
ERF
RF
ERF
SHH
BE QUIET!
CANS EVERYWHERE INSIDE. BUT DID I HAVE A RIGHT TO WALTZ IN AND HELP MYSELF?
door wide open. Nobody home.
Yes! I'VE HIT THE MOTHER LODE!
THIS SURE WAS SOME PARTY!
I GOT THIS--
NO PROBLEM
AND, IF ANYONE WERE TO ASK, I'LL JUST SAY "I'M JASON'S MOM." THERE'S BOUND TO BE A JASON AROUND HERE SOMEWHERE.
NOBODY ASKED. NOBODY NOTICED ME HAULING OUT 6 BAGS OF CANS!
SSH, DOG! QUIET!!
ERF
ERF
I'M TRYING TO GET AWAY WITH A CRIME HERE.
ERF
AND SO IT GOES FOR THE INVISIBLE LADY--
WE PAY CASH FOR CANS $
SIR!
STEP OVER HERE AND I'LL GET YOU WEIGHED.
ARR!
CT

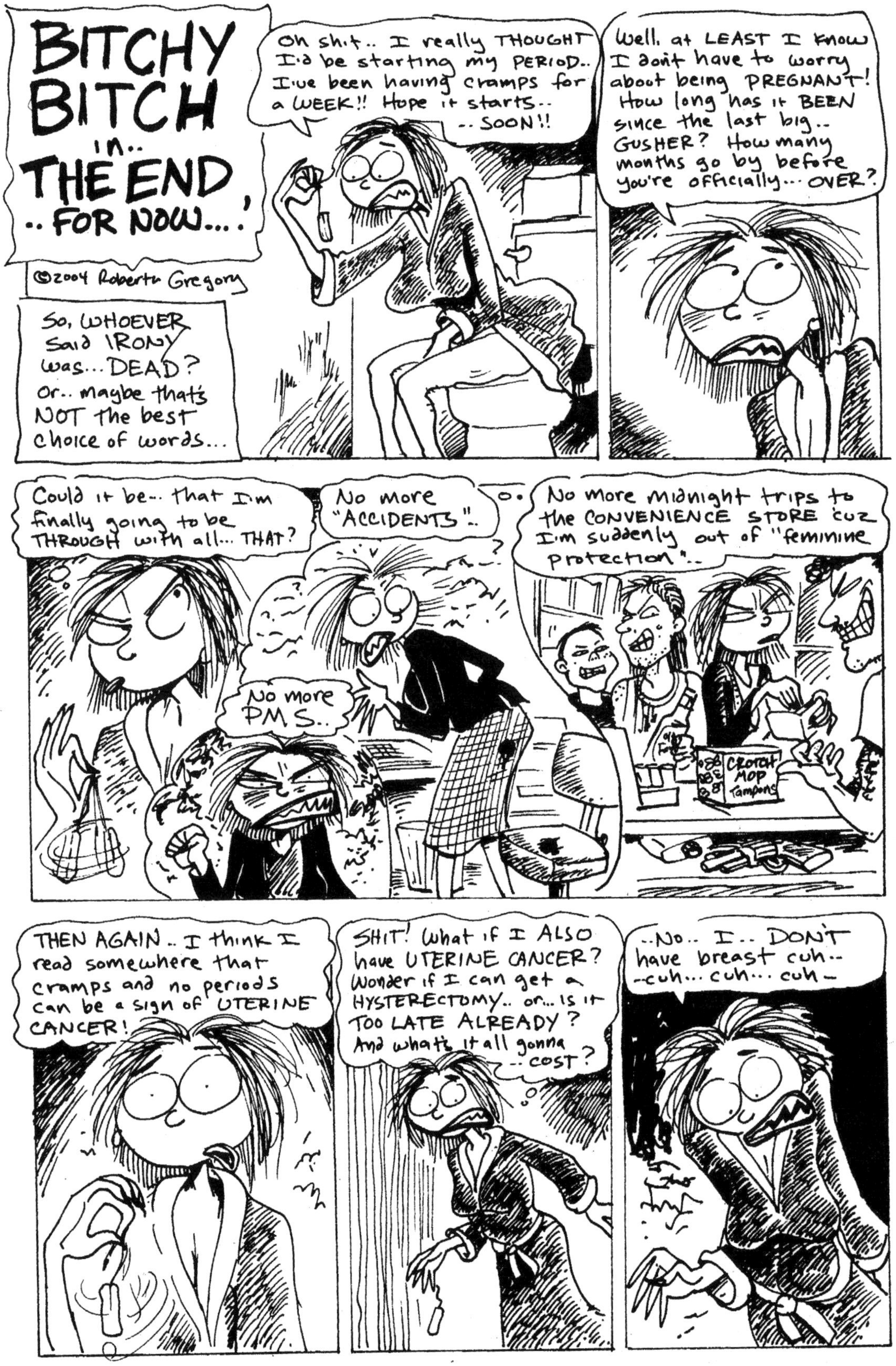
BITCHY BITCH in.. THE END ..FOR NOW....'
©2004 Roberta Gregory
So, WHOEVER said IRONY was... DEAD? or.. maybe that's NOT the best choice of words...
Oh shit.. I really THOUGHT I'd be starting my PERIOD.. I've been having cramps for a WEEK!! Hope it starts.. --SOON!!
Well, at LEAST I know I don't have to worry about being PREGNANT! How long has it BEEN since the last big.. GUSHER? How many months go by before you're officially... OVER?
Could it be-- that I'm finally going to be THROUGH with all... THAT?
No more "ACCIDENTS"..
No more P.M.S..
No more midnight trips to the CONVENIENCE STORE 'cuz I'm suddenly out of "feminine protection"..
CROTCH MOP Tampons
THEN AGAIN.. I think I read somewhere that cramps and no periods can be a sign of UTERINE CANCER!
SHIT! What if I ALSO have UTERINE CANCER? Wonder if I can get a HYSTERECTOMY.. or... is it TOO LATE ALREADY? And what's it all gonna --cost?
--No.. I.. DON'T have breast cuh-- --cuh... cuh... cuh--

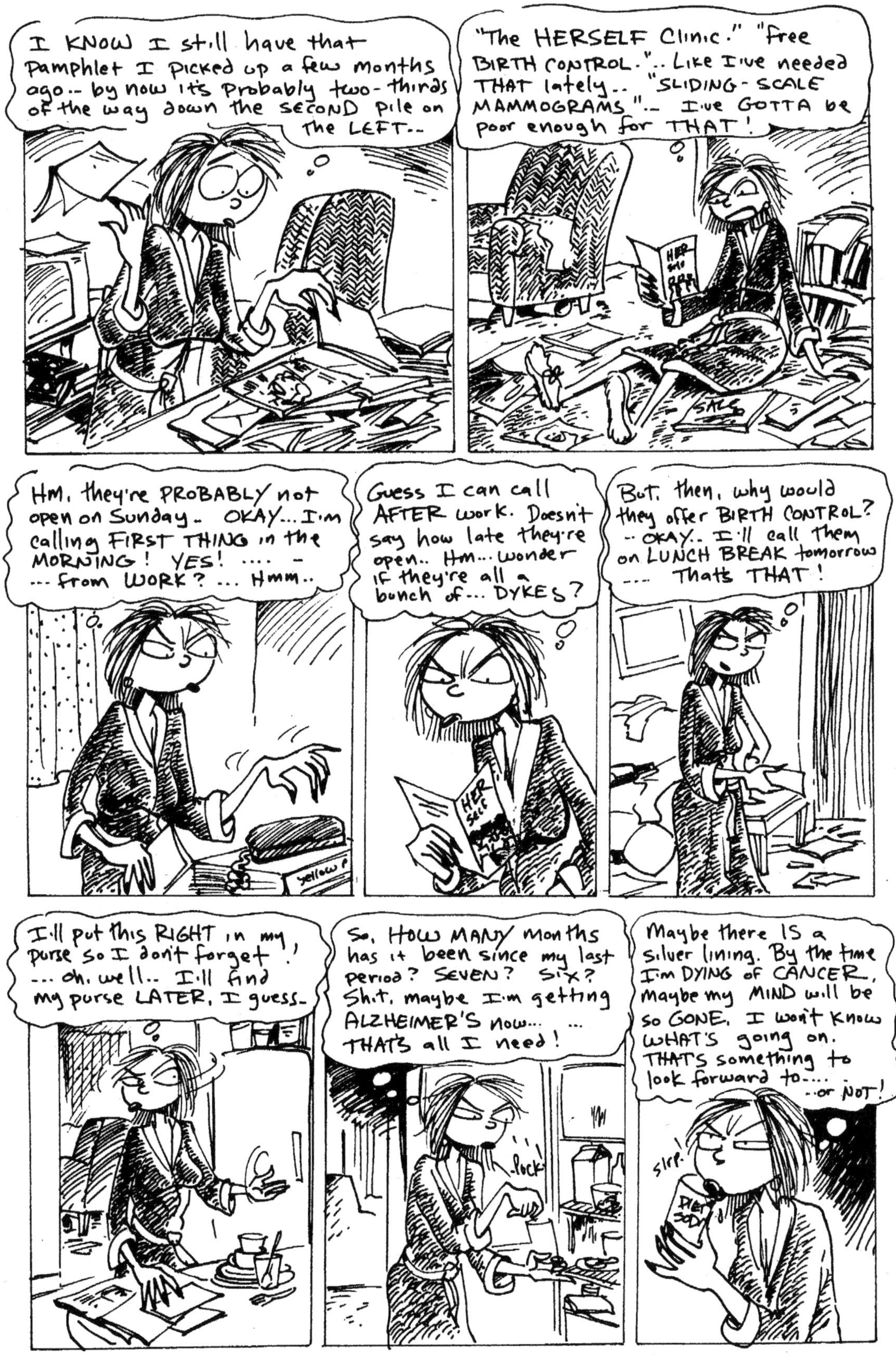
I KNOW I still have that pamphlet I picked up a few months ago.. by now it's probably two-thirds of the way down the SECOND pile on the LEFT..
"The HERSELF Clinic." "Free BIRTH CONTROL.".. Like I've needed THAT lately.. "SLIDING-SCALE MAMMOGRAMS".. I've GOTTA be poor enough for THAT!
HER SELF
SALE
Hm. they're PROBABLY not open on Sunday.. OKAY... I'm calling FIRST THING in the MORNING! YES! .... from WORK? ... Hmm..
yellow P
Guess I can call AFTER work. Doesn't say how late they're open.. Hm... wonder if they're all a bunch of... DYKES?
HER SELF
But, then, why would they offer BIRTH CONTROL? -- OKAY.. I'll call them on LUNCH BREAK tomorrow --- That's THAT!
I'll put this RIGHT in my purse so I don't forget! ... oh, well.. I'll find my purse LATER, I guess..
So, HOW MANY months has it been since my last period? SEVEN? Six? Shit, maybe I'm getting ALZHEIMER'S now... ... THAT'S all I need!
pock
Maybe there IS a silver lining. By the time I'm DYING of CANCER, maybe my MIND will be so GONE, I won't know WHAT'S going on. THAT'S something to look forward to.... ..or NOT!
slrp
DIET SODA

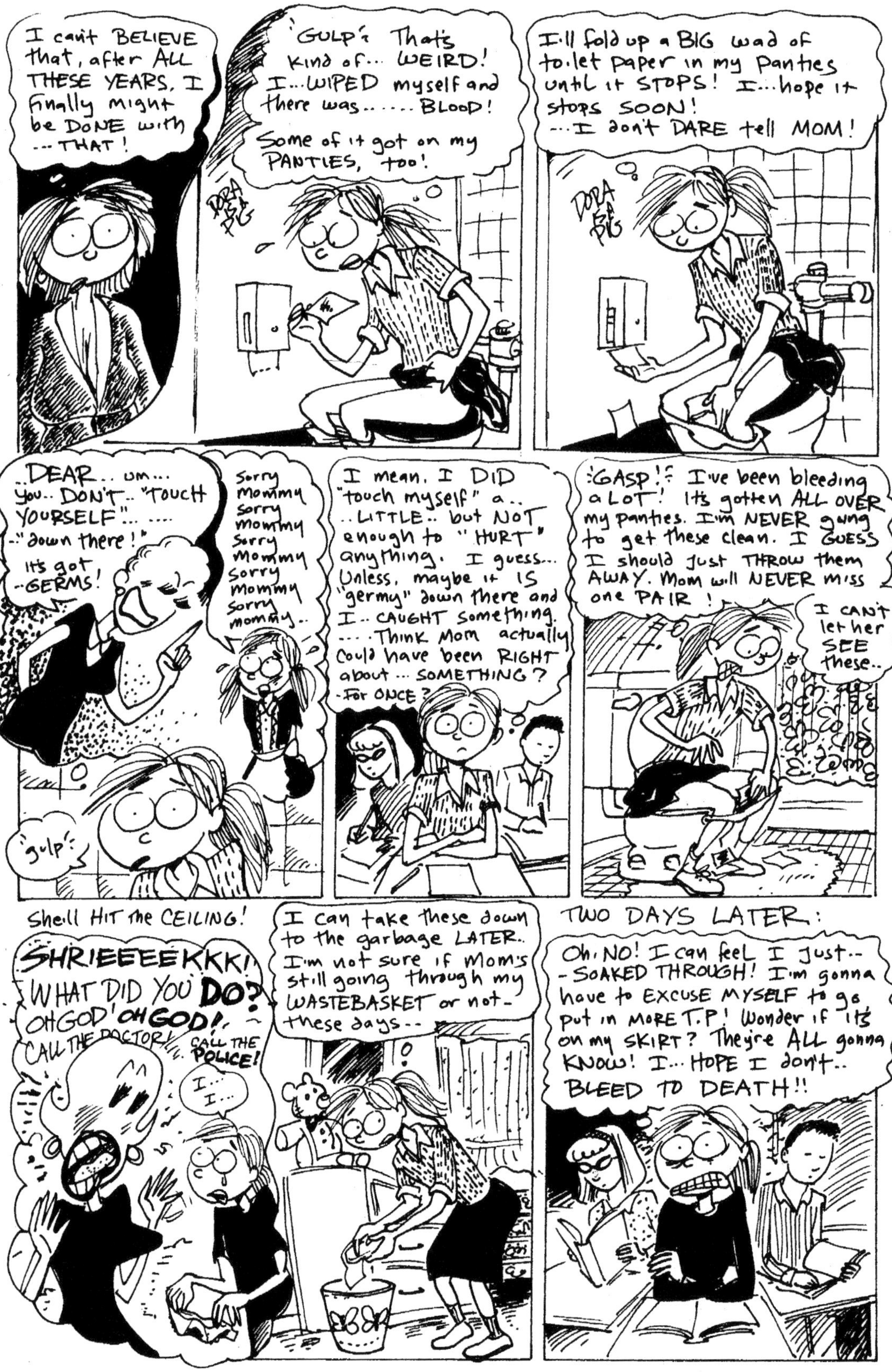
I can't BELIEVE that, after ALL THESE YEARS, I finally might be DONE with ---THAT!
GULP! That's kind of... WEIRD! I...WIPED myself and there was...... BLOOD!
Some of it got on my PANTIES, too!
DORA IS A PIG
I'll fold up a BIG wad of toilet paper in my panties until it STOPS! I...hope it stops SOON!
---I don't DARE tell MOM!
DORA IS A PIG
..DEAR.. um... you.. DON'T.. "TOUCH YOURSELF"... .... .."down there!" It's got GERMS!
sorry mommy sorry mommy sorry mommy sorry mommy sorry mommy..
gulp!
I mean, I DID "touch myself" a.. ..LITTLE.. but NOT enough to "HURT" anything. I guess... Unless, maybe it IS "germy" down there and I... CAUGHT something. ....Think Mom actually could have been RIGHT about... SOMETHING? -For ONCE?
GASP! I've been bleeding a LOT! It's gotten ALL OVER my panties. I'm NEVER going to get these clean. I GUESS I should just THROW them AWAY. Mom will NEVER miss one PAIR!
I CAN'T let her SEE these..
She'll HIT the CEILING!
SHRIEEEEKKK! WHAT DID YOU DO? OH GOD! OH GOD! CALL THE DOCTOR! CALL THE POLICE!
I... I...
I can take these down to the garbage LATER.. I'm not sure if Mom's still going through my WASTEBASKET or not-these days--
TWO DAYS LATER:
Oh, NO! I can feel I just.. -SOAKED THROUGH! I'm gonna have to EXCUSE MYSELF to go put in MORE T.P! Wonder if it's on my SKIRT? They're ALL gonna KNOW! I... HOPE I don't.. BLEED TO DEATH!!

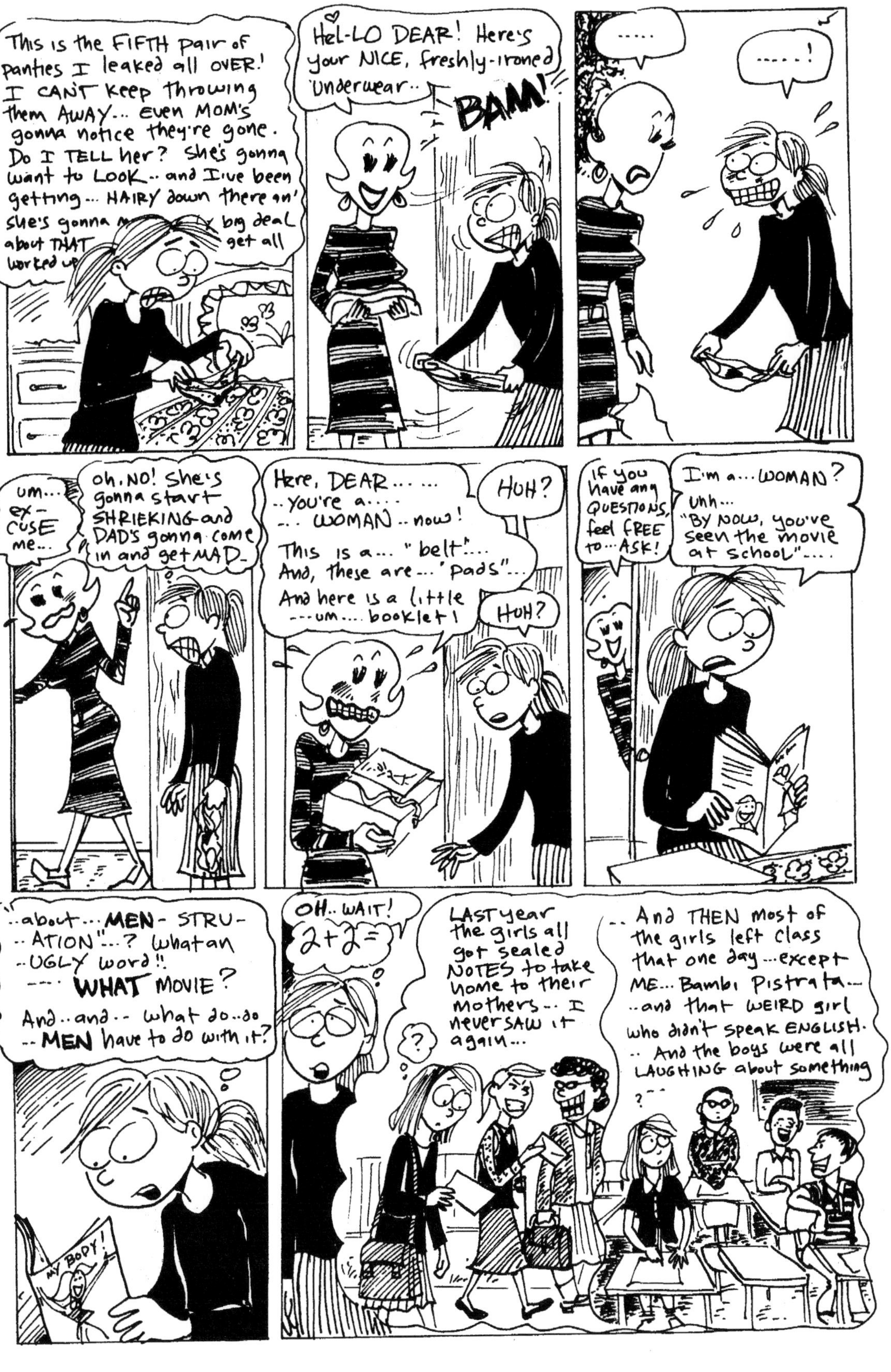
This is the FIFTH pair of panties I leaked all OVER! I CAN'T keep throwing them AWAY... Even MOM's gonna notice they're gone. Do I TELL her? She's gonna want to LOOK.. and I've been getting... HAIRY down there an' she's gonna m big deal about THAT get all worked u
Hel-LO DEAR! Here's your NICE, freshly-ironed underwear..
BAM!
.....
.....!
um... ex-CUSE me...
oh, NO! She's gonna start SHRIEKING and DAD'S gonna come in and get MAD_
Here, DEAR...... ..you're a.... ... WOMAN .. now! This is a... "belt"... And, these are..."pads"... And here is a little ---um.... booklet!
HUH?
HUH?
If you have any QUESTIONS, feel FREE to... ASK!
I'm a... WOMAN? uhh... "By now, you've seen the movie at school"....
MY BODY!
..about... MEN- STRU- ..ATION"...? What an ..UGLY word!! ---.. WHAT MOVIE? And..and.. what do..do ..MEN have to do with it?
OH.. WAIT! 2+2=
?
LAST year the girls all got sealed NOTES to take home to their mothers.. I never SAW it again...
..And THEN most of the girls left class that one day...except ME... Bambi Pistrata.... ..and that WEIRD girl who didn't speak ENGLISH. .. And the boys were all LAUGHING about something ?--

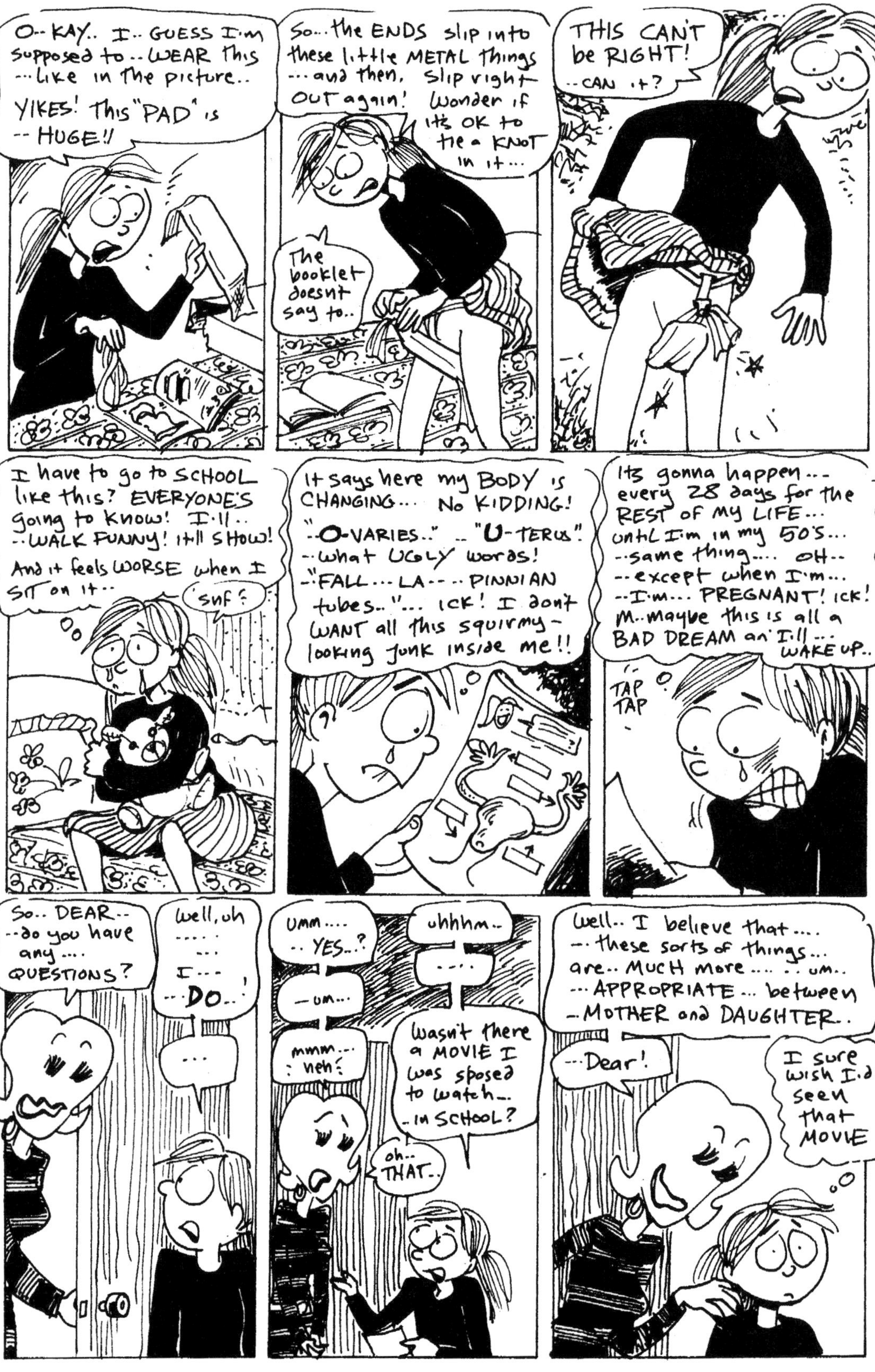
O-- KAY.. I.. GUESS I'm supposed to -- WEAR this --- like in the picture.. YIKES! This "PAD" is -- HUGE!!
So... the ENDS slip into these little METAL things --- and then, slip right OUT again! Wonder if it's OK to tie a KNOT in it...
The booklet doesn't say to..
THIS CAN'T be RIGHT! --CAN it?
I have to go to SCHOOL like this? EVERYONE'S going to know! I-ll.. --WALK FUNNY! it'll SHOW! And it feels WORSE when I SIT on it--
snf!
It says here my BODY is CHANGING... No KIDDING! "O-VARIES.." .. "U-TERUS". --what UGLY words! --"FALL...LA---PINNIAN tubes.."... ICK! I don't WANT all this squirmy-looking junk inside me!!
It's gonna happen--- every 28 days for the REST of MY LIFE... until I'm in my 50's... --same thing.... OH-- --except when I'm... --I'm... PREGNANT! ick! M..maybe this is all a BAD DREAM an' I'll ... WAKE UP..
TAP TAP
So.. DEAR-- --do you have any.... QUESTIONS?
Well, uh .... I--- --DO..
...
umm.... .. YES..?
uhhhm..
...
--um..
mmm... : neh?
Wasn't there a MOVIE I was sposed to watch.. ..in SCHOOL?
oh.. THAT..
Well.. I believe that.... --these sorts of things... are.. MUCH more.... ..um.. ---APPROPRIATE... between --MOTHER and DAUGHTER..
--Dear!
I sure wish I'd seen that MOVIE..

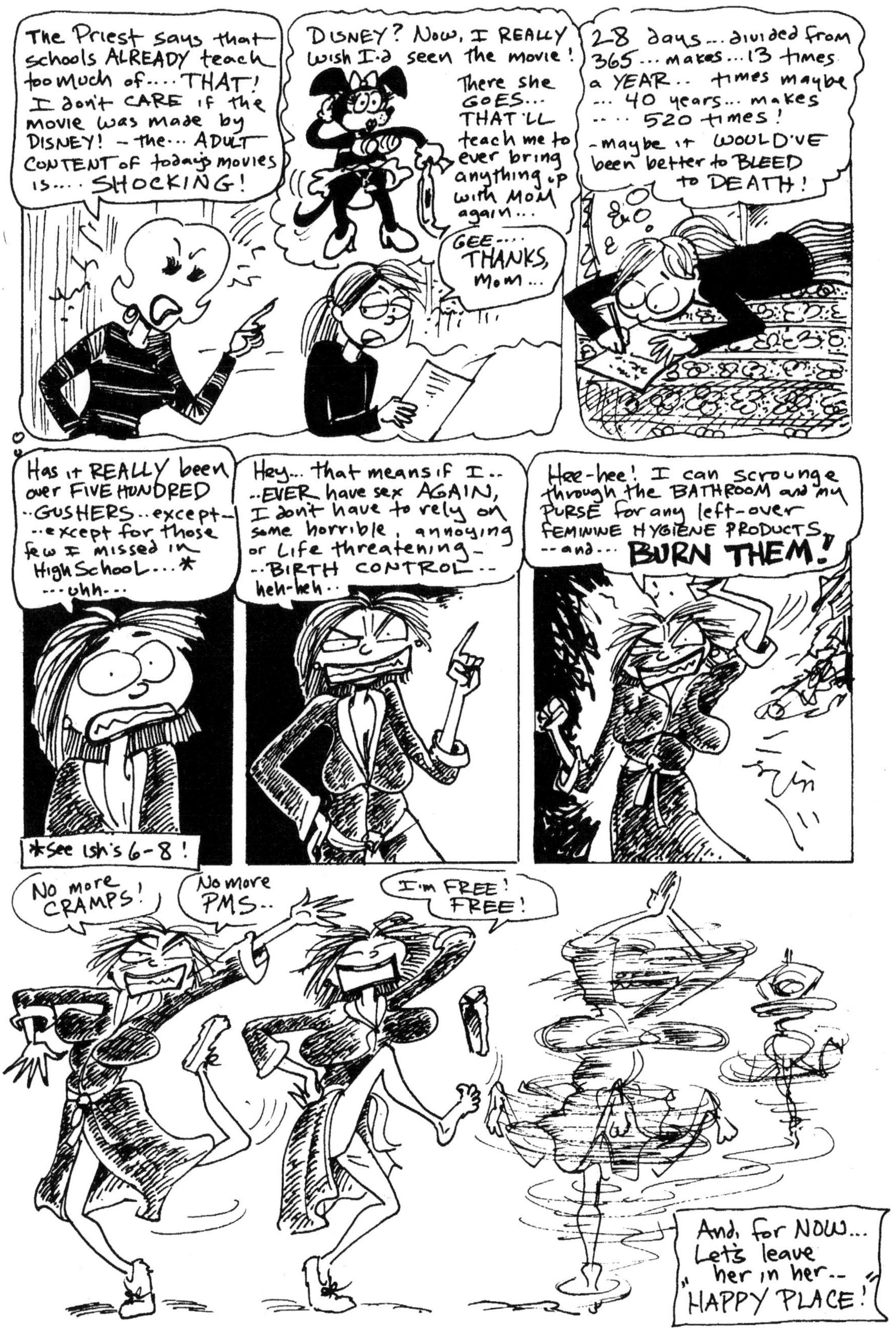

The Priest says that schools ALREADY teach too much of.... THAT! I don't CARE if the movie was made by DISNEY! — the... ADULT CONTENT of today's movies is.... SHOCKING!
DISNEY? Now, I REALLY wish I'd seen the movie!
There she GOES... THAT'LL teach me to ever bring anything up with MOM again...
GEE.... THANKS, MOM...
28 days... divided from 365... makes... 13 times a YEAR.. times maybe ... 40 years... makes ... 520 times!
- maybe it WOULD'VE been better to BLEED to DEATH!
Has it REALLY been over FIVE HUNDRED ..GUSHERS.. except- --except for those few I missed in High School...* ---uhh---
*See ish's 6-8!
Hey... that means if I.. ..EVER have sex AGAIN, I don't have to rely on some horrible, annoying or Life threatening- --BIRTH CONTROL-- heh-heh..
Hee-hee! I can scrounge through the BATHROOM and my PURSE for any left-over FEMININE HYGIENE PRODUCTS, --and... BURN THEM!
No more CRAMPS!
No more PMS..
I'm FREE! FREE!
And, for NOW... Let's leave her in her.. "HAPPY PLACE!"

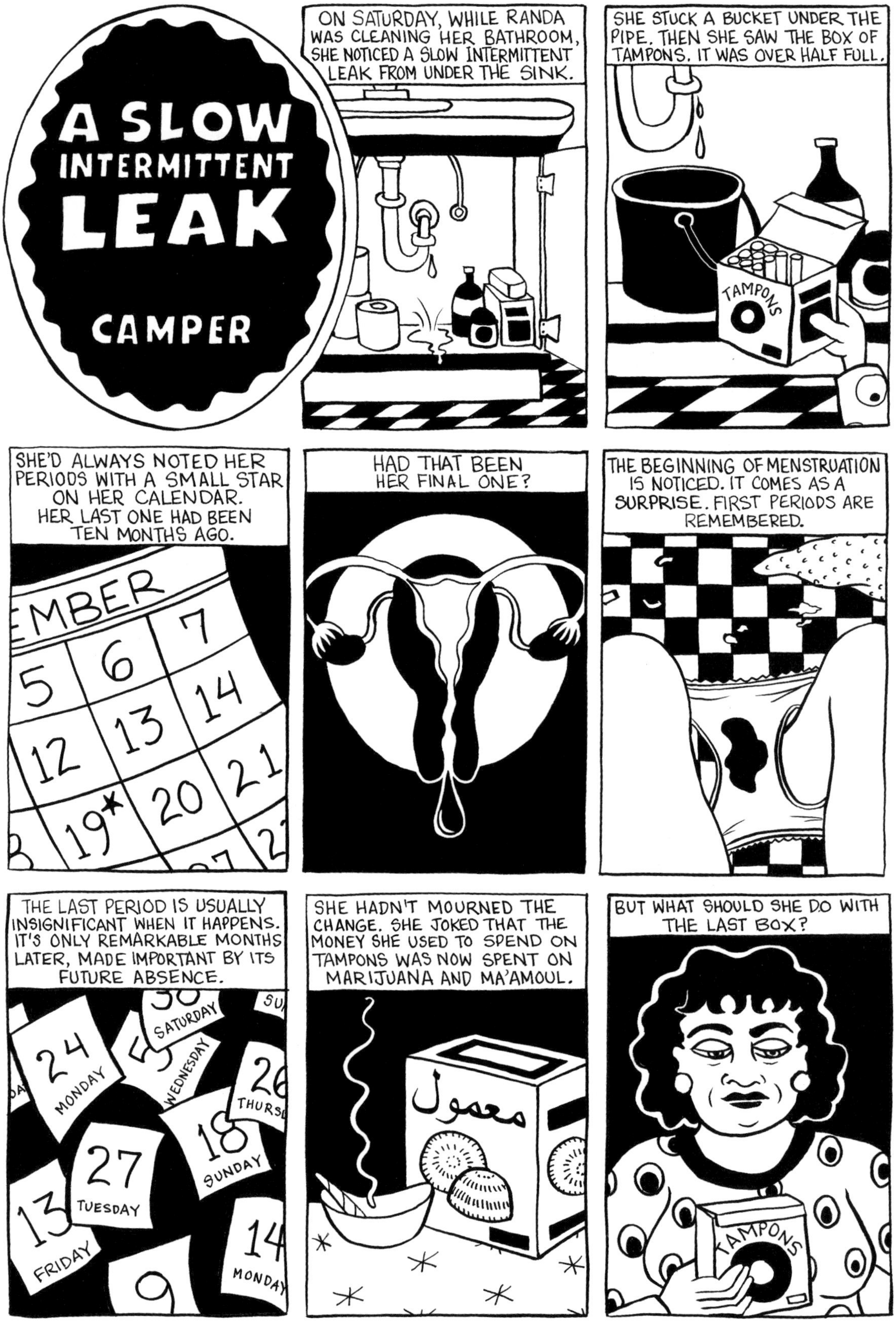
A SLOW INTERMITTENT LEAK
CAMPER
ON SATURDAY, WHILE RANDA WAS CLEANING HER BATHROOM, SHE NOTICED A SLOW INTERMITTENT LEAK FROM UNDER THE SINK.
SHE STUCK A BUCKET UNDER THE PIPE. THEN SHE SAW THE BOX OF TAMPONS. IT WAS OVER HALF FULL.
TAMPONS
SHE'D ALWAYS NOTED HER PERIODS WITH A SMALL STAR ON HER CALENDAR. HER LAST ONE HAD BEEN TEN MONTHS AGO.
EMBER
5 6 7
12 13 14
19* 20 21
HAD THAT BEEN HER FINAL ONE?
THE BEGINNING OF MENSTRUATION IS NOTICED. IT COMES AS A SURPRISE. FIRST PERIODS ARE REMEMBERED.
THE LAST PERIOD IS USUALLY INSIGNIFICANT WHEN IT HAPPENS. IT'S ONLY REMARKABLE MONTHS LATER, MADE IMPORTANT BY ITS FUTURE ABSENCE.
24 MONDAY
SATURDAY
WEDNESDAY
26 THURS
18 SUNDAY
27 TUESDAY
13 FRIDAY
14 MONDAY
SHE HADN'T MOURNED THE CHANGE. SHE JOKED THAT THE MONEY SHE USED TO SPEND ON TAMPONS WAS NOW SPENT ON MARIJUANA AND MA'AMOUL.
معمول
BUT WHAT SHOULD SHE DO WITH THE LAST BOX?
TAMPONS

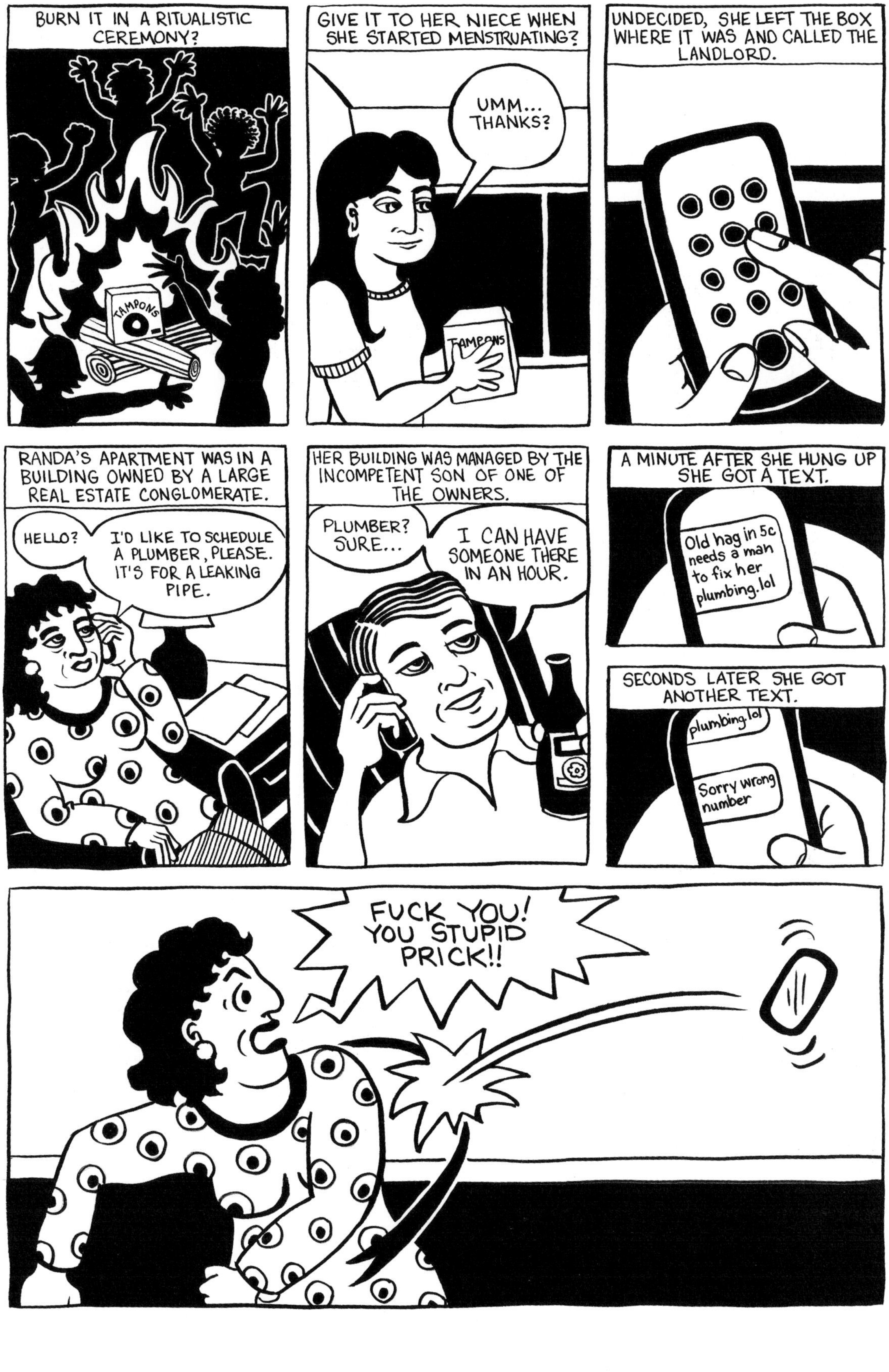
BURN IT IN A RITUALISTIC CEREMONY?
TAMPONS
GIVE IT TO HER NIECE WHEN SHE STARTED MENSTRUATING?
UMM... THANKS?
TAMPONS
UNDECIDED, SHE LEFT THE BOX WHERE IT WAS AND CALLED THE LANDLORD.
RANDA'S APARTMENT WAS IN A BUILDING OWNED BY A LARGE REAL ESTATE CONGLOMERATE.
HELLO?
I'D LIKE TO SCHEDULE A PLUMBER, PLEASE. IT'S FOR A LEAKING PIPE.
HER BUILDING WAS MANAGED BY THE INCOMPETENT SON OF ONE OF THE OWNERS.
PLUMBER? SURE...
I CAN HAVE SOMEONE THERE IN AN HOUR.
A MINUTE AFTER SHE HUNG UP SHE GOT A TEXT.
Old hag in 5c needs a man to fix her plumbing. lol
SECONDS LATER SHE GOT ANOTHER TEXT.
plumbing. lol
Sorry wrong number
FUCK YOU! YOU STUPID PRICK!!

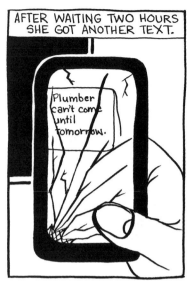

AFTER WAITING TWO HOURS SHE GOT ANOTHER TEXT.

Plumber can't come until tomorrow.

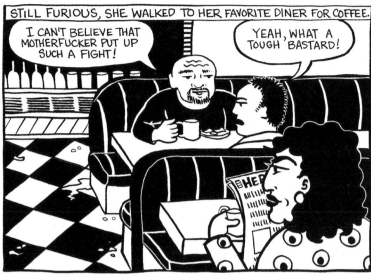

STILL FURIOUS, SHE WALKED TO HER FAVORITE DINER FOR COFFEE.

I CAN'T BELIEVE THAT MOTHERFUCKER PUT UP SUCH A FIGHT!

YEAH, WHAT A TOUGH BASTARD!

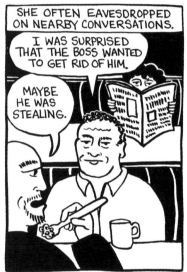

SHE OFTEN EAVESDROPPED ON NEARBY CONVERSATIONS.

I WAS SURPRISED THAT THE BOSS WANTED TO GET RID OF HIM.

MAYBE HE WAS STEALING.

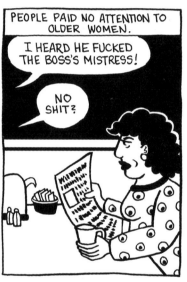

PEOPLE PAID NO ATTENTION TO OLDER WOMEN.

I HEARD HE FUCKED THE BOSS'S MISTRESS!

NO SHIT?

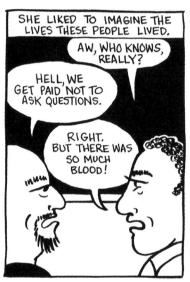

SHE LIKED TO IMAGINE THE LIVES THESE PEOPLE LIVED.

AW, WHO KNOWS, REALLY?

HELL, WE GET PAID NOT TO ASK QUESTIONS.

RIGHT. BUT THERE WAS SO MUCH BLOOD!

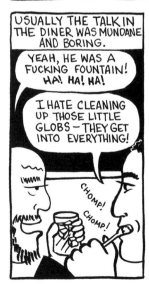

USUALLY THE TALK IN THE DINER WAS MUNDANE AND BORING.

YEAH, HE WAS A FUCKING FOUNTAIN! HA! HA! HA!

I HATE CLEANING UP THOSE LITTLE GLOBS—THEY GET INTO EVERYTHING!

CHOMP! CHOMP!

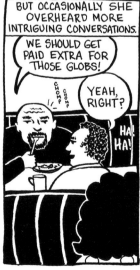

BUT OCCASIONALLY SHE OVERHEARD MORE INTRIGUING CONVERSATIONS.

WE SHOULD GET PAID EXTRA FOR THOSE GLOBS!

YEAH, RIGHT?

CHOMP CHOMP

HA! HA!

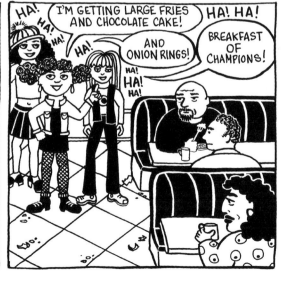

HA! HA! HA!

I'M GETTING LARGE FRIES AND CHOCOLATE CAKE!

HA! HA!

AND ONION RINGS!

BREAKFAST OF CHAMPIONS!

HA! HA! HA!

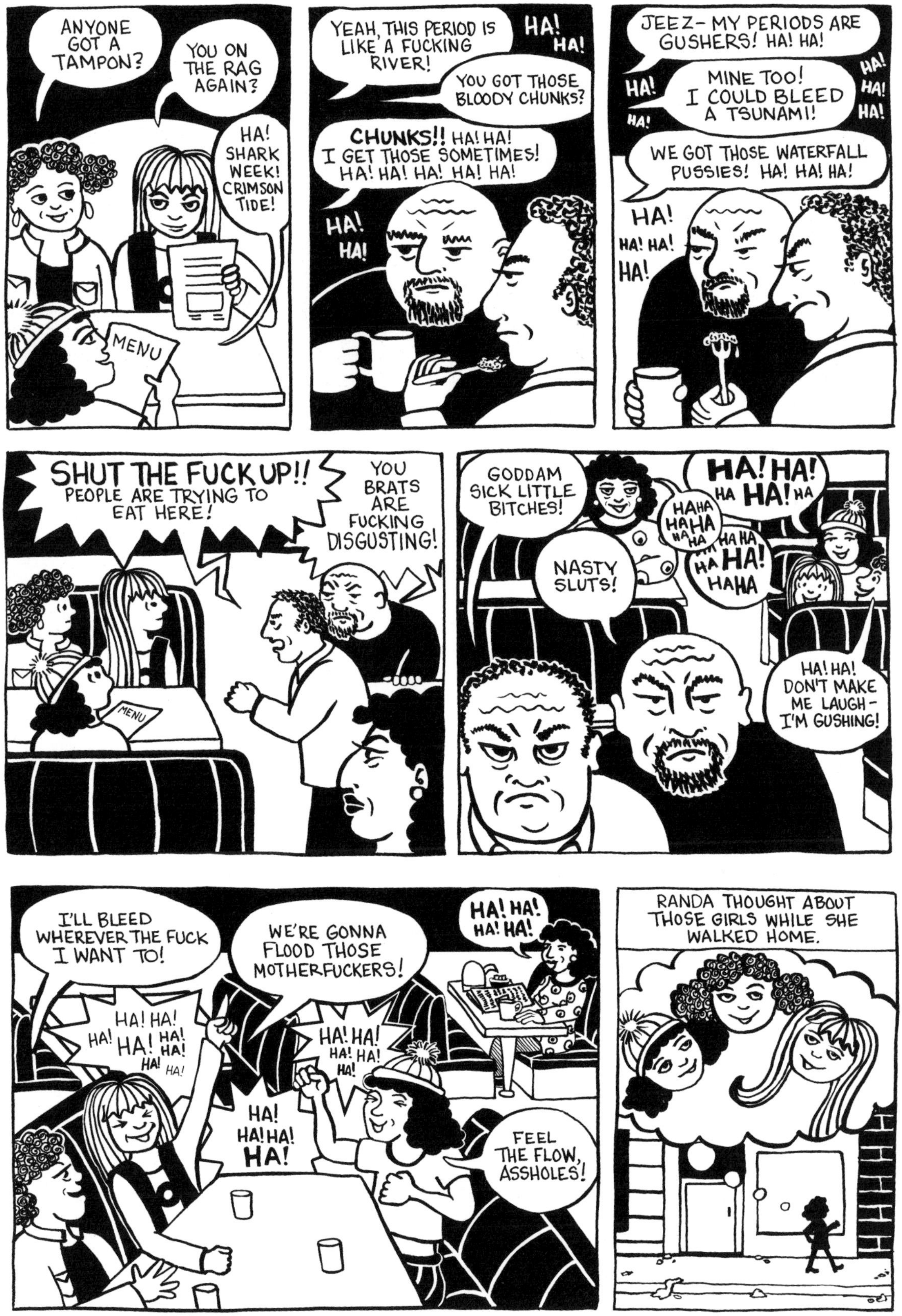
ANYONE GOT A TAMPON?
YOU ON THE RAG AGAIN?
HA! SHARK WEEK! CRIMSON TIDE!
MENU
YEAH, THIS PERIOD IS LIKE A FUCKING RIVER!
HA! HA!
YOU GOT THOSE BLOODY CHUNKS?
CHUNKS!! HA! HA! I GET THOSE SOMETIMES! HA! HA! HA! HA! HA!
HA! HA!
JEEZ- MY PERIODS ARE GUSHERS! HA! HA!
HA! HA!
MINE TOO! I COULD BLEED A TSUNAMI!
HA! HA! HA!
WE GOT THOSE WATERFALL PUSSIES! HA! HA! HA!
HA! HA! HA! HA!
SHUT THE FUCK UP!! PEOPLE ARE TRYING TO EAT HERE!
YOU BRATS ARE FUCKING DISGUSTING!
MENU
GODDAM SICK LITTLE BITCHES!
NASTY SLUTS!
HA! HA! HA HA! HA
HA HA HA HA HA HA
HA HA HA HA! HA HA
HA! HA! DON'T MAKE ME LAUGH- I'M GUSHING!
I'LL BLEED WHEREVER THE FUCK I WANT TO!
HA! HA! HA! HA! HA! HA! HA! HA!
WE'RE GONNA FLOOD THOSE MOTHERFUCKERS!
HA! HA! HA! HA! HA! HA!
HA! HA! HA! HA!
HA! HA! HA! HA!
FEEL THE FLOW, ASSHOLES!
RANDA THOUGHT ABOUT THOSE GIRLS WHILE SHE WALKED HOME.

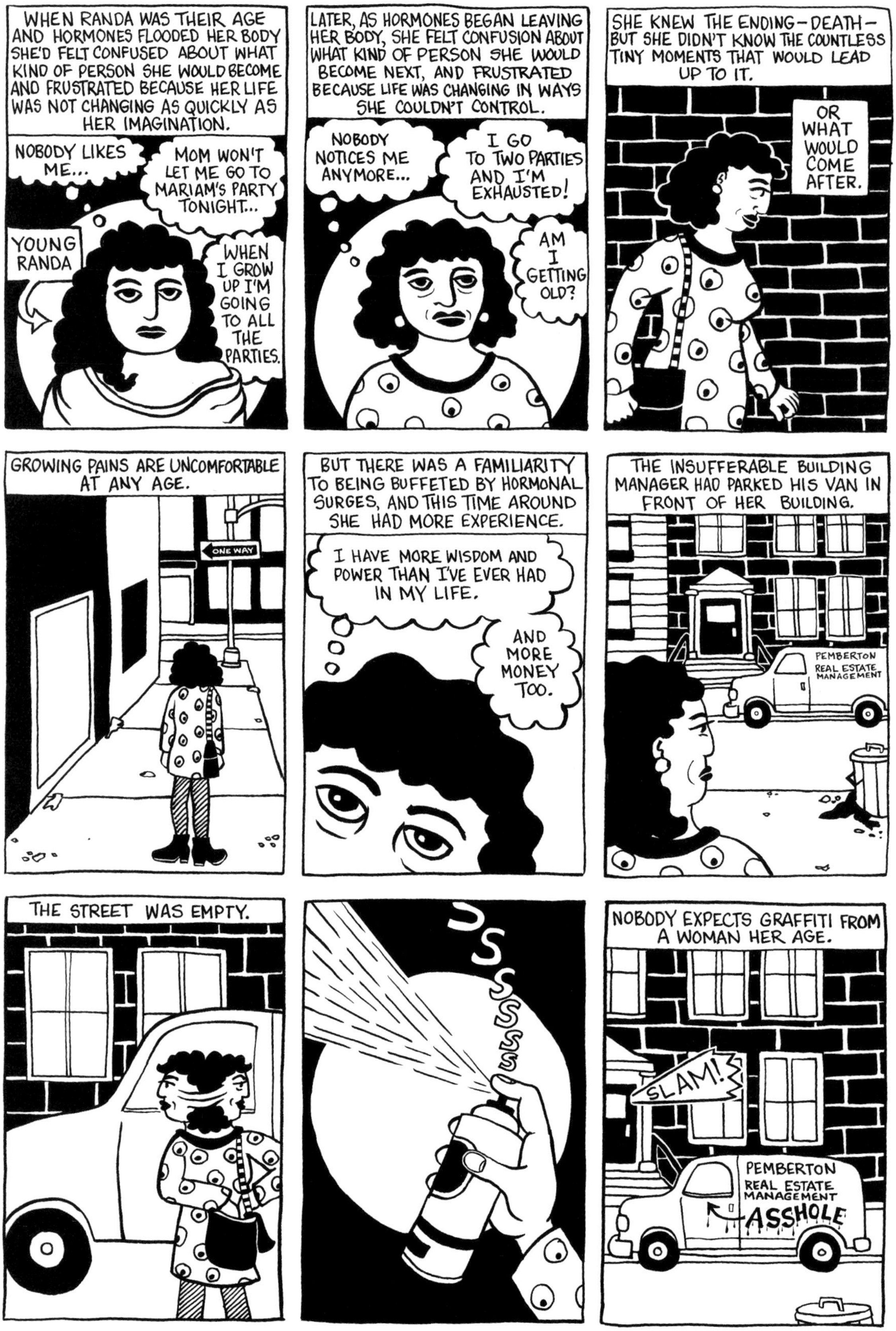
WHEN RANDA WAS THEIR AGE AND HORMONES FLOODED HER BODY SHE'D FELT CONFUSED ABOUT WHAT KIND OF PERSON SHE WOULD BECOME AND FRUSTRATED BECAUSE HER LIFE WAS NOT CHANGING AS QUICKLY AS HER IMAGINATION.
NOBODY LIKES ME...
MOM WON'T LET ME GO TO MARIAM'S PARTY TONIGHT...
YOUNG RANDA
WHEN I GROW UP I'M GOING TO ALL THE PARTIES.
LATER, AS HORMONES BEGAN LEAVING HER BODY, SHE FELT CONFUSION ABOUT WHAT KIND OF PERSON SHE WOULD BECOME NEXT, AND FRUSTRATED BECAUSE LIFE WAS CHANGING IN WAYS SHE COULDN'T CONTROL.
NOBODY NOTICES ME ANYMORE...
I GO TO TWO PARTIES AND I'M EXHAUSTED!
AM I GETTING OLD?
SHE KNEW THE ENDING–DEATH–BUT SHE DIDN'T KNOW THE COUNTLESS TINY MOMENTS THAT WOULD LEAD UP TO IT.
OR WHAT WOULD COME AFTER.
GROWING PAINS ARE UNCOMFORTABLE AT ANY AGE.
ONE WAY
BUT THERE WAS A FAMILIARITY TO BEING BUFFETED BY HORMONAL SURGES, AND THIS TIME AROUND SHE HAD MORE EXPERIENCE.
I HAVE MORE WISDOM AND POWER THAN I'VE EVER HAD IN MY LIFE.
AND MORE MONEY TOO.
THE INSUFFERABLE BUILDING MANAGER HAD PARKED HIS VAN IN FRONT OF HER BUILDING.
PEMBERTON REAL ESTATE MANAGEMENT
THE STREET WAS EMPTY.
SSSSSS
NOBODY EXPECTS GRAFFITI FROM A WOMAN HER AGE.
SLAM!
PEMBERTON REAL ESTATE MANAGEMENT
ASSHOLE

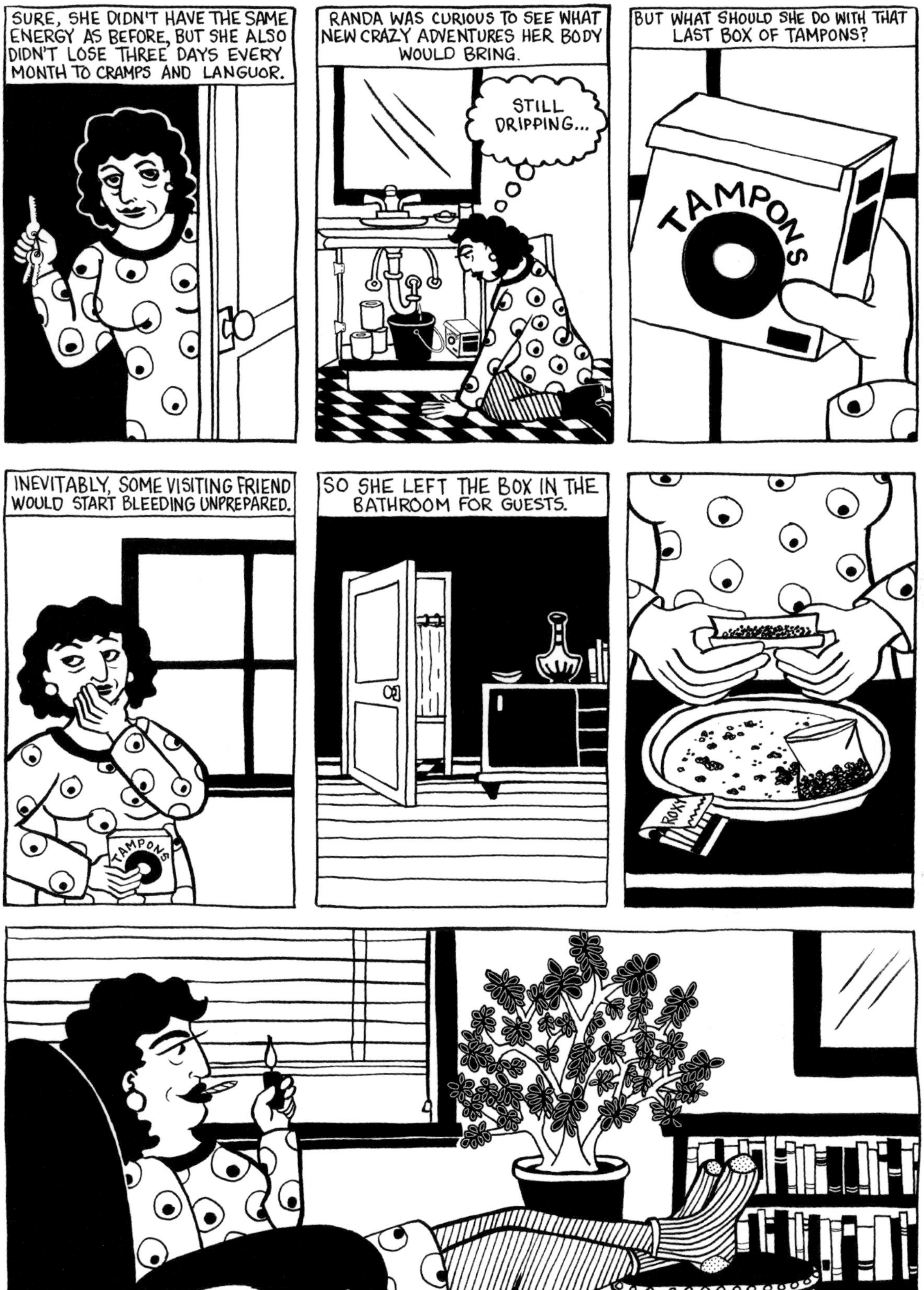
SURE, SHE DIDN'T HAVE THE SAME ENERGY AS BEFORE, BUT SHE ALSO DIDN'T LOSE THREE DAYS EVERY MONTH TO CRAMPS AND LANGUOR.
RANDA WAS CURIOUS TO SEE WHAT NEW CRAZY ADVENTURES HER BODY WOULD BRING.
STILL DRIPPING...
BUT WHAT SHOULD SHE DO WITH THAT LAST BOX OF TAMPONS?
TAMPONS
INEVITABLY, SOME VISITING FRIEND WOULD START BLEEDING UNPREPARED.
TAMPONS
SO SHE LEFT THE BOX IN THE BATHROOM FOR GUESTS.
ROXY

A Slow Intermittent Leak

Jennifer Camper

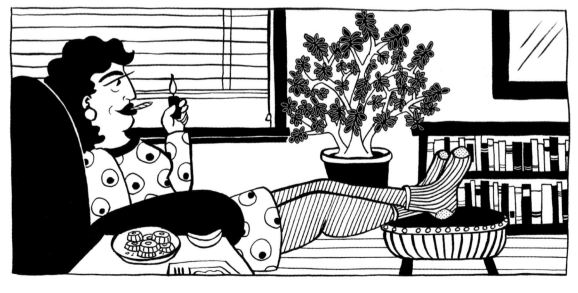

Nicola Streeten

2.14am-4.43am

tomorrow no not
is sun
I could get up and look
that article
I don't feel the slight
oh bloody hell here we
if this is
Another
oh god the summer is nearly over already
I should
I must start writing
was completed
that was

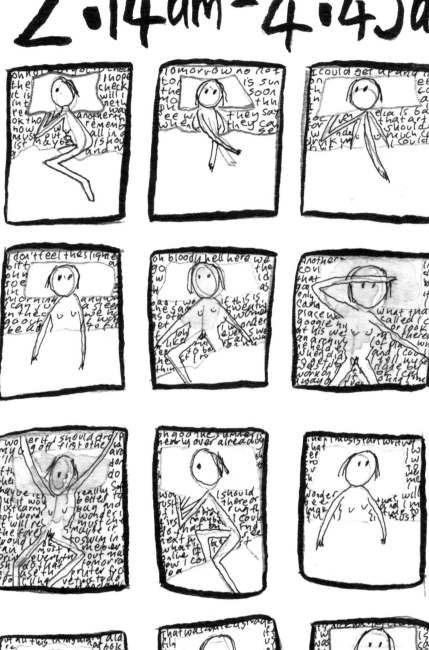

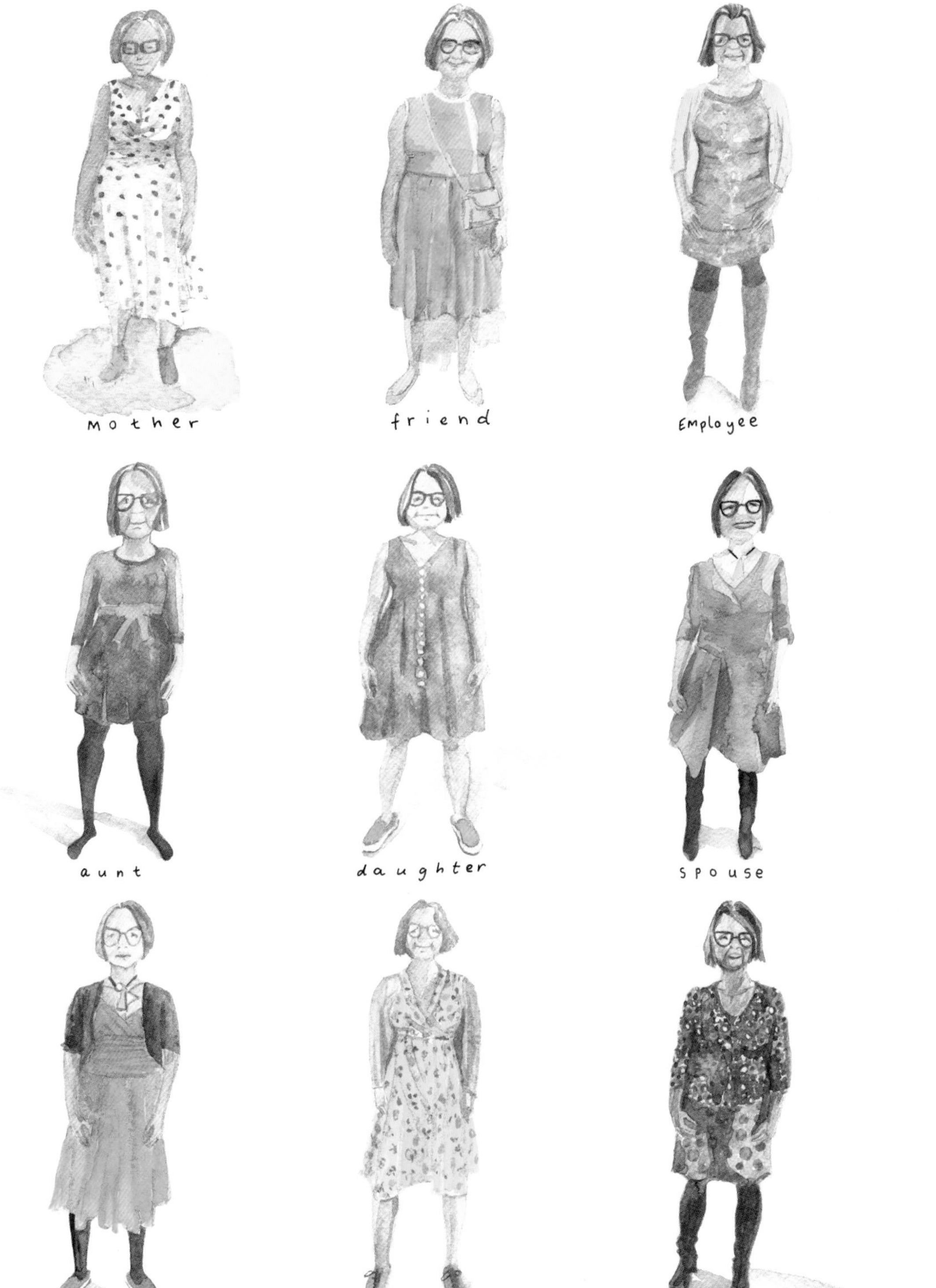
mother
friend
Employee
aunt
daughter
spouse
teacher
sister
neighbour

Any Day Now

by Ajuan Mance

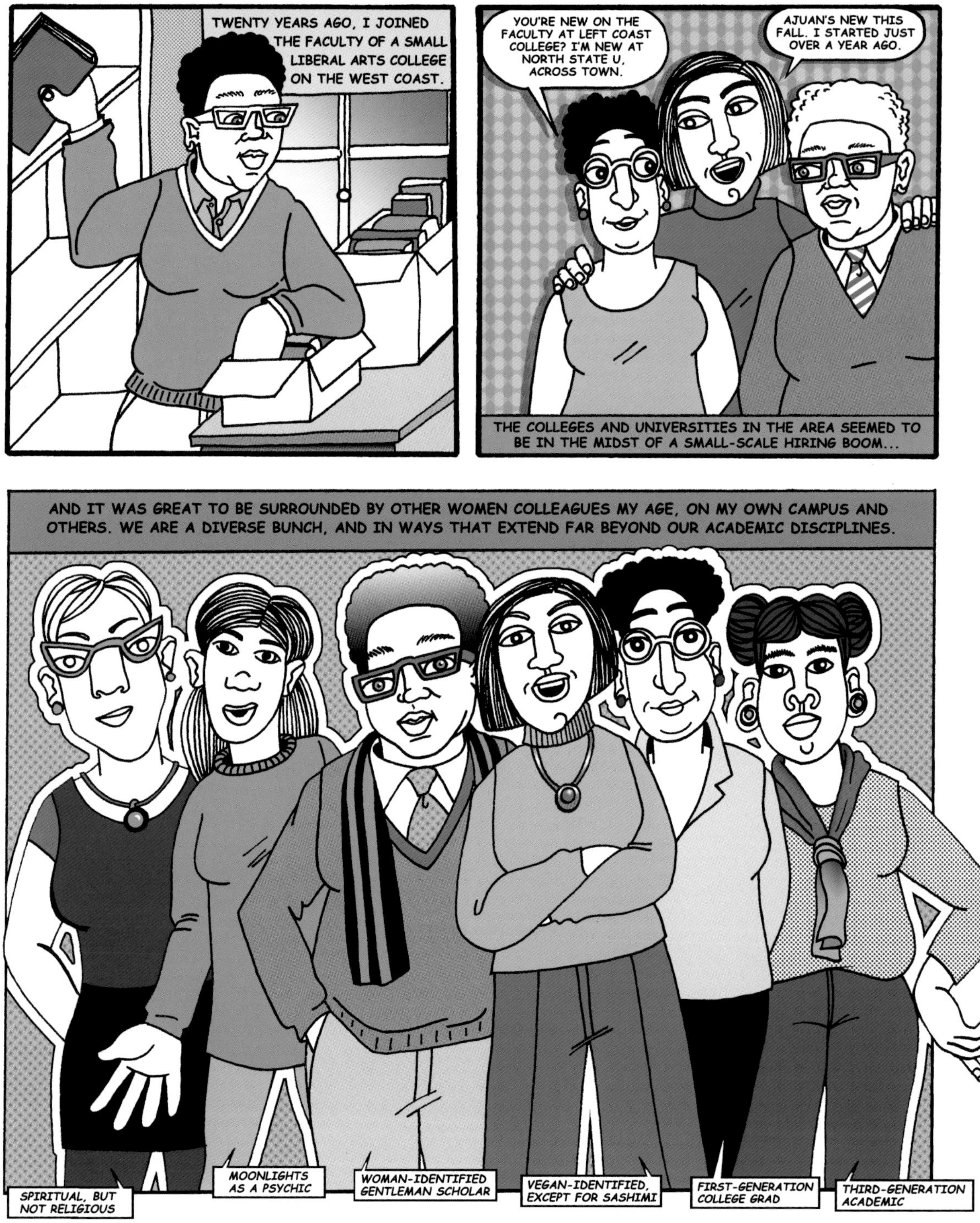
TWENTY YEARS AGO, I JOINED THE FACULTY OF A SMALL LIBERAL ARTS COLLEGE ON THE WEST COAST.
YOU'RE NEW ON THE FACULTY AT LEFT COAST COLLEGE? I'M NEW AT NORTH STATE U, ACROSS TOWN.
AJUAN'S NEW THIS FALL. I STARTED JUST OVER A YEAR AGO.
THE COLLEGES AND UNIVERSITIES IN THE AREA SEEMED TO BE IN THE MIDST OF A SMALL-SCALE HIRING BOOM...
AND IT WAS GREAT TO BE SURROUNDED BY OTHER WOMEN COLLEAGUES MY AGE, ON MY OWN CAMPUS AND OTHERS. WE ARE A DIVERSE BUNCH, AND IN WAYS THAT EXTEND FAR BEYOND OUR ACADEMIC DISCIPLINES.
SPIRITUAL, BUT NOT RELIGIOUS
MOONLIGHTS AS A PSYCHIC
WOMAN-IDENTIFIED GENTLEMAN SCHOLAR
VEGAN-IDENTIFIED, EXCEPT FOR SASHIMI
FIRST-GENERATION COLLEGE GRAD
THIRD-GENERATION ACADEMIC

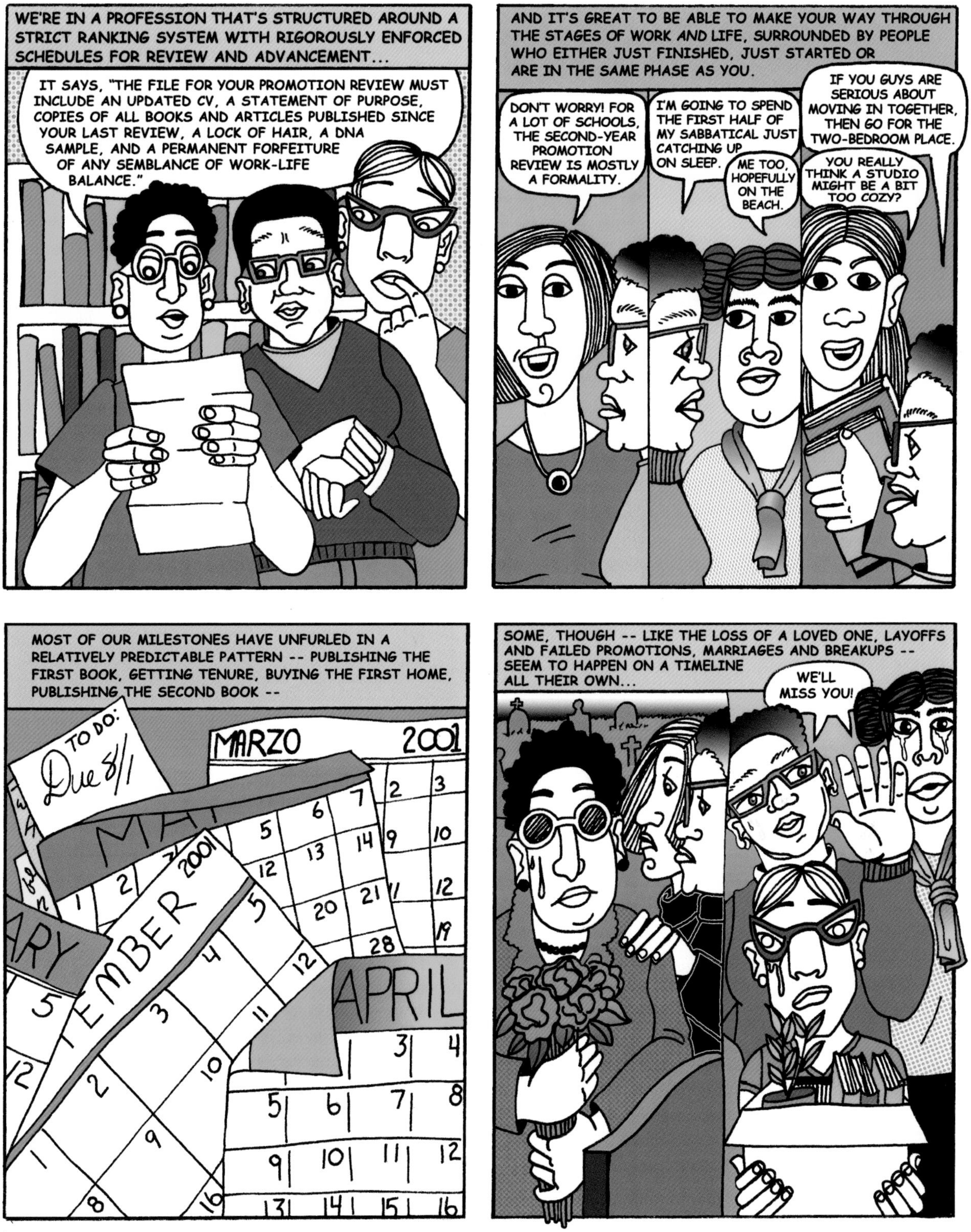
WE'RE IN A PROFESSION THAT'S STRUCTURED AROUND A STRICT RANKING SYSTEM WITH RIGOROUSLY ENFORCED SCHEDULES FOR REVIEW AND ADVANCEMENT...
IT SAYS, "THE FILE FOR YOUR PROMOTION REVIEW MUST INCLUDE AN UPDATED CV, A STATEMENT OF PURPOSE, COPIES OF ALL BOOKS AND ARTICLES PUBLISHED SINCE YOUR LAST REVIEW, A LOCK OF HAIR, A DNA SAMPLE, AND A PERMANENT FORFEITURE OF ANY SEMBLANCE OF WORK-LIFE BALANCE."
AND IT'S GREAT TO BE ABLE TO MAKE YOUR WAY THROUGH THE STAGES OF WORK AND LIFE, SURROUNDED BY PEOPLE WHO EITHER JUST FINISHED, JUST STARTED OR ARE IN THE SAME PHASE AS YOU.
DON'T WORRY! FOR A LOT OF SCHOOLS, THE SECOND-YEAR PROMOTION REVIEW IS MOSTLY A FORMALITY.
I'M GOING TO SPEND THE FIRST HALF OF MY SABBATICAL JUST CATCHING UP ON SLEEP.
ME TOO, HOPEFULLY ON THE BEACH.
IF YOU GUYS ARE SERIOUS ABOUT MOVING IN TOGETHER, THEN GO FOR THE TWO-BEDROOM PLACE.
YOU REALLY THINK A STUDIO MIGHT BE A BIT TOO COZY?
MOST OF OUR MILESTONES HAVE UNFURLED IN A RELATIVELY PREDICTABLE PATTERN -- PUBLISHING THE FIRST BOOK, GETTING TENURE, BUYING THE FIRST HOME, PUBLISHING THE SECOND BOOK --
TO DO:
Due 8/1
MARZO 2001
2001
APRIL
SOME, THOUGH -- LIKE THE LOSS OF A LOVED ONE, LAYOFFS AND FAILED PROMOTIONS, MARRIAGES AND BREAKUPS -- SEEM TO HAPPEN ON A TIMELINE ALL THEIR OWN...
WE'LL MISS YOU!

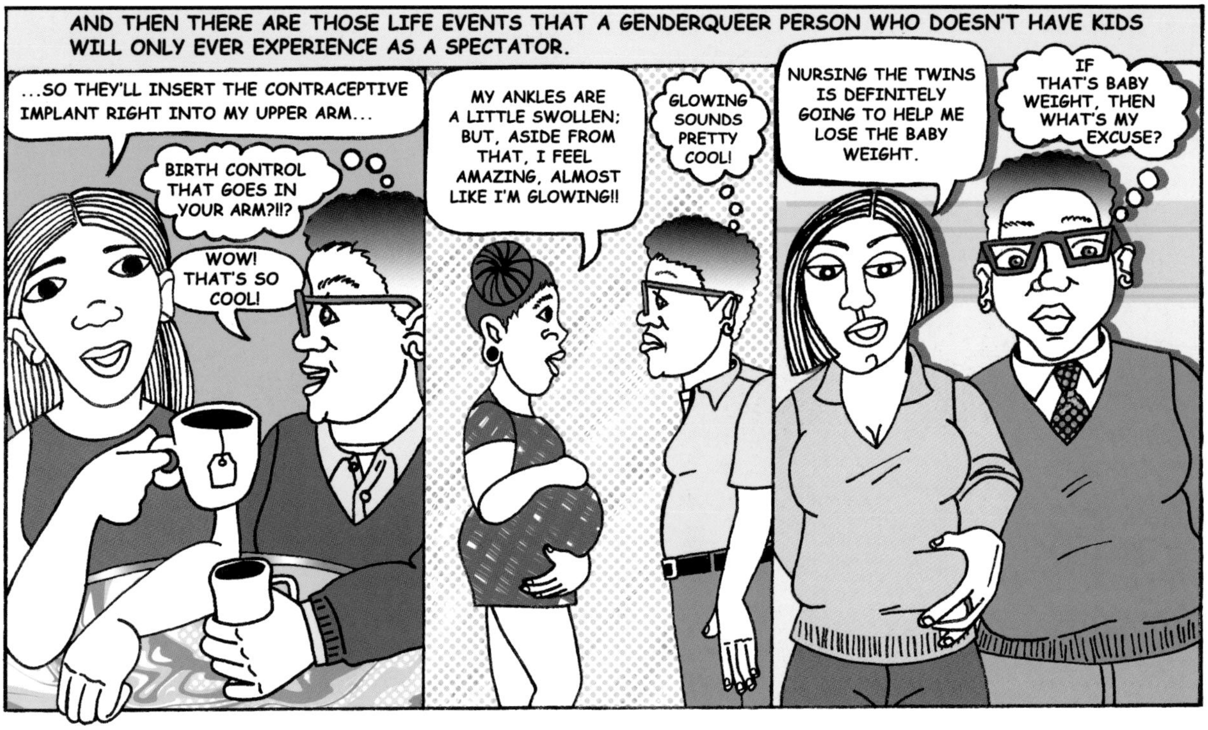
AND THEN THERE ARE THOSE LIFE EVENTS THAT A GENDERQUEER PERSON WHO DOESN'T HAVE KIDS WILL ONLY EVER EXPERIENCE AS A SPECTATOR.
...SO THEY'LL INSERT THE CONTRACEPTIVE IMPLANT RIGHT INTO MY UPPER ARM...
BIRTH CONTROL THAT GOES IN YOUR ARM?!!?
WOW! THAT'S SO COOL!
MY ANKLES ARE A LITTLE SWOLLEN; BUT, ASIDE FROM THAT, I FEEL AMAZING, ALMOST LIKE I'M GLOWING!!
GLOWING SOUNDS PRETTY COOL!
NURSING THE TWINS IS DEFINITELY GOING TO HELP ME LOSE THE BABY WEIGHT.
IF THAT'S BABY WEIGHT, THEN WHAT'S MY EXCUSE?

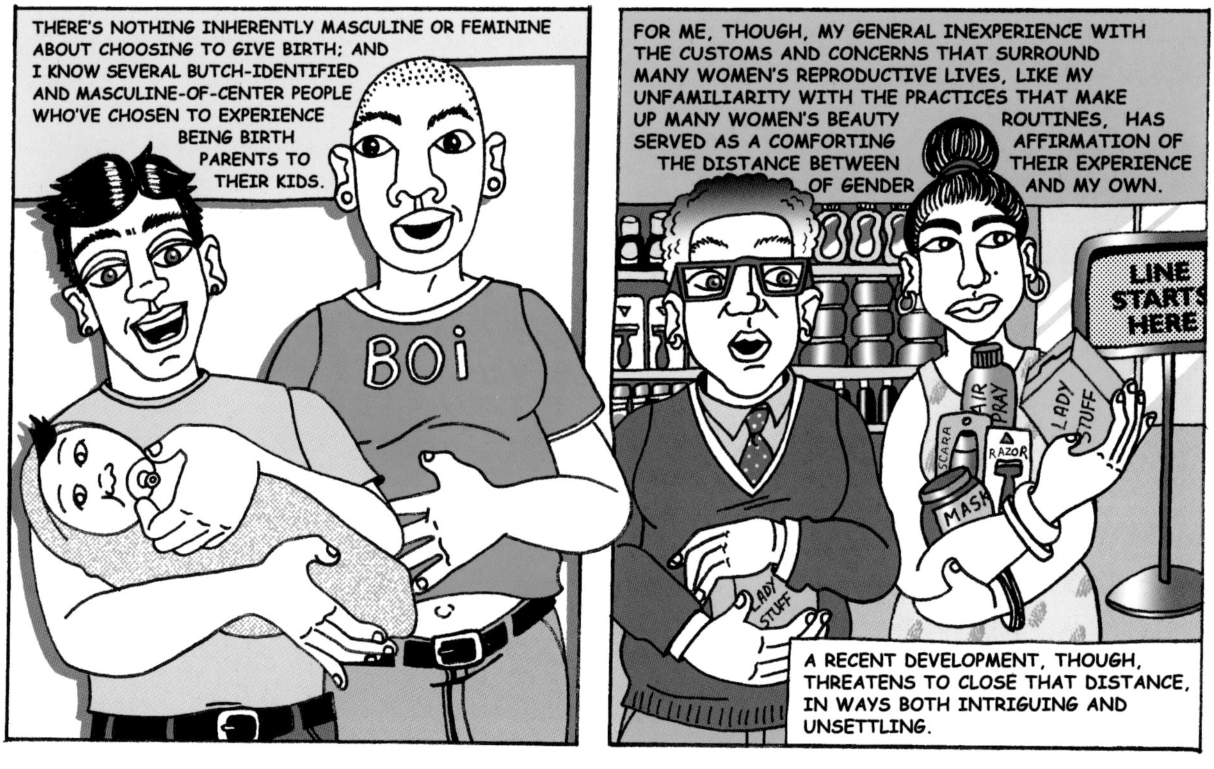
THERE'S NOTHING INHERENTLY MASCULINE OR FEMININE ABOUT CHOOSING TO GIVE BIRTH; AND I KNOW SEVERAL BUTCH-IDENTIFIED AND MASCULINE-OF-CENTER PEOPLE WHO'VE CHOSEN TO EXPERIENCE BEING BIRTH PARENTS TO THEIR KIDS.
BOi
FOR ME, THOUGH, MY GENERAL INEXPERIENCE WITH THE CUSTOMS AND CONCERNS THAT SURROUND MANY WOMEN'S REPRODUCTIVE LIVES, LIKE MY UNFAMILIARITY WITH THE PRACTICES THAT MAKE UP MANY WOMEN'S BEAUTY ROUTINES, HAS SERVED AS A COMFORTING AFFIRMATION OF THE DISTANCE BETWEEN THEIR EXPERIENCE OF GENDER AND MY OWN.
LINE STARTS HERE
LADY STUFF
RAZOR
MASK
LADY STUFF
A RECENT DEVELOPMENT, THOUGH, THREATENS TO CLOSE THAT DISTANCE, IN WAYS BOTH INTRIGUING AND UNSETTLING.

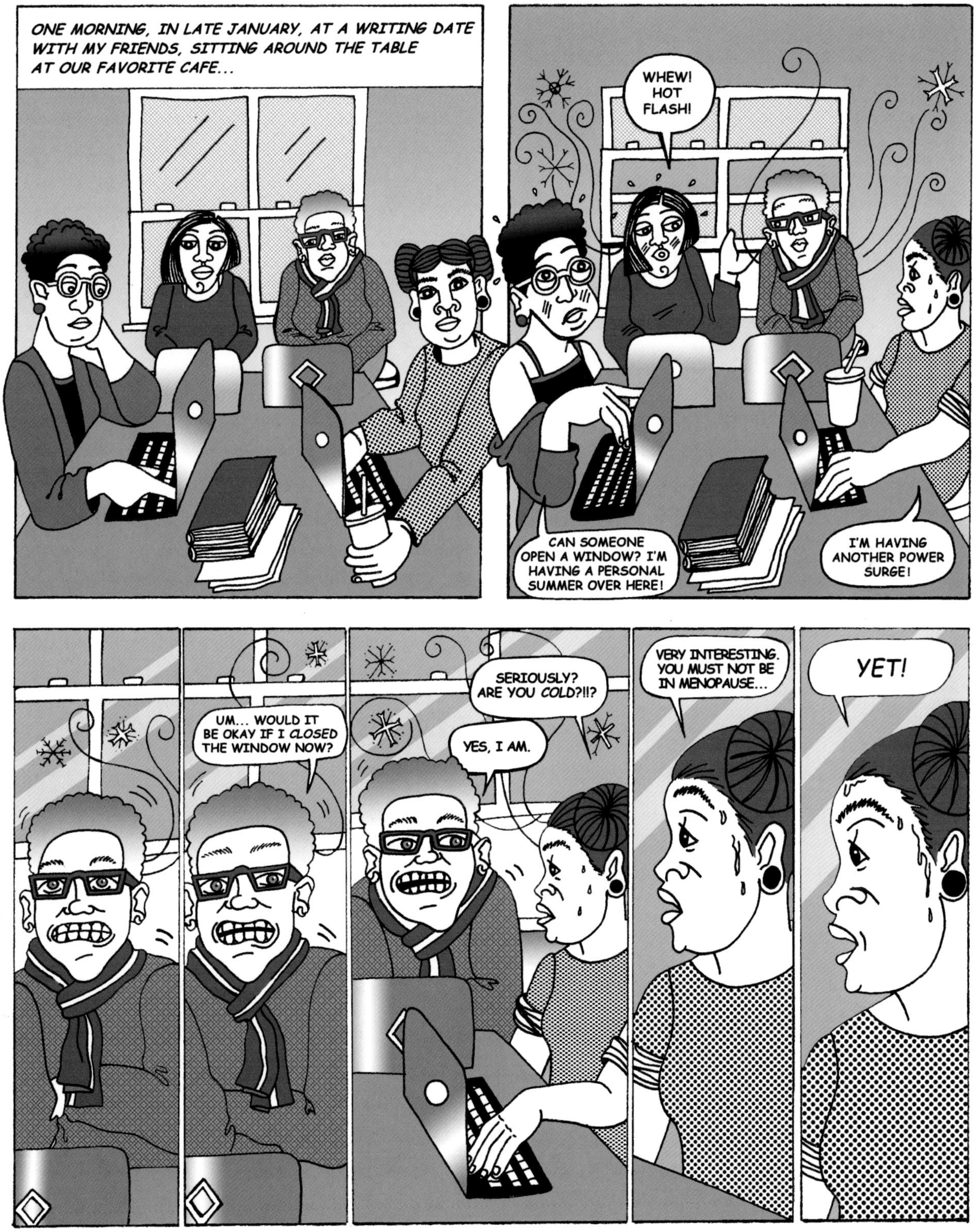
ONE MORNING, IN LATE JANUARY, AT A WRITING DATE WITH MY FRIENDS, SITTING AROUND THE TABLE AT OUR FAVORITE CAFE...
WHEW! HOT FLASH!
CAN SOMEONE OPEN A WINDOW? I'M HAVING A PERSONAL SUMMER OVER HERE!
I'M HAVING ANOTHER POWER SURGE!
UM... WOULD IT BE OKAY IF I CLOSED THE WINDOW NOW?
SERIOUSLY? ARE YOU COLD?!!?
YES, I AM.
VERY INTERESTING. YOU MUST NOT BE IN MENOPAUSE...
YET!

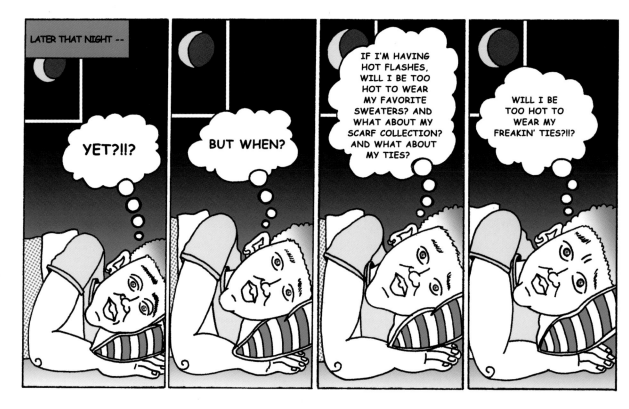

LATER THAT NIGHT --

YET?!!?

BUT WHEN?

IF I'M HAVING HOT FLASHES, WILL I BE TOO HOT TO WEAR MY FAVORITE SWEATERS? AND WHAT ABOUT MY SCARF COLLECTION? AND WHAT ABOUT MY TIES?

WILL I BE TOO HOT TO WEAR MY FREAKIN' TIES?!!?

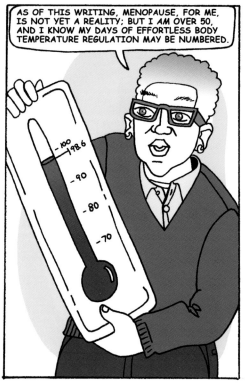

AS OF THIS WRITING, MENOPAUSE, FOR ME, IS NOT YET A REALITY; BUT I AM OVER 50, AND I KNOW MY DAYS OF EFFORTLESS BODY TEMPERATURE REGULATION MAY BE NUMBERED.

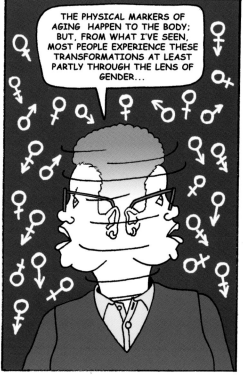

THE PHYSICAL MARKERS OF AGING HAPPEN TO THE BODY; BUT, FROM WHAT I'VE SEEN, MOST PEOPLE EXPERIENCE THESE TRANSFORMATIONS AT LEAST PARTLY THROUGH THE LENS OF GENDER...

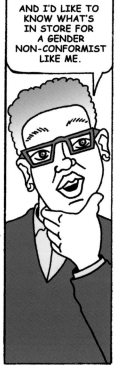

AND I'D LIKE TO KNOW WHAT'S IN STORE FOR A GENDER NON-CONFORMIST LIKE ME.

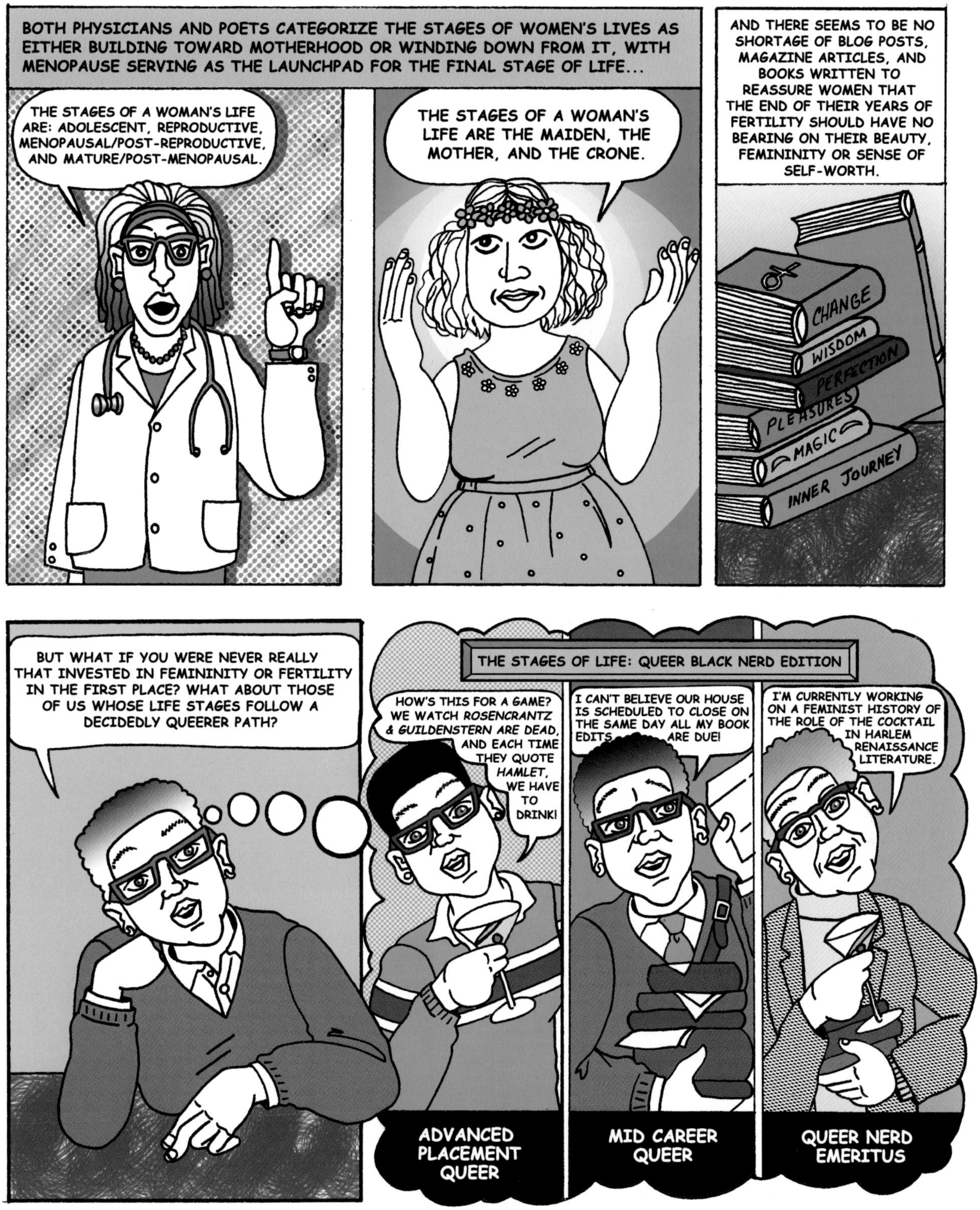
BOTH PHYSICIANS AND POETS CATEGORIZE THE STAGES OF WOMEN'S LIVES AS EITHER BUILDING TOWARD MOTHERHOOD OR WINDING DOWN FROM IT, WITH MENOPAUSE SERVING AS THE LAUNCHPAD FOR THE FINAL STAGE OF LIFE...
THE STAGES OF A WOMAN'S LIFE ARE: ADOLESCENT, REPRODUCTIVE, MENOPAUSAL/POST-REPRODUCTIVE, AND MATURE/POST-MENOPAUSAL.
THE STAGES OF A WOMAN'S LIFE ARE THE MAIDEN, THE MOTHER, AND THE CRONE.
AND THERE SEEMS TO BE NO SHORTAGE OF BLOG POSTS, MAGAZINE ARTICLES, AND BOOKS WRITTEN TO REASSURE WOMEN THAT THE END OF THEIR YEARS OF FERTILITY SHOULD HAVE NO BEARING ON THEIR BEAUTY, FEMININITY OR SENSE OF SELF-WORTH.
CHANGE
WISDOM
PERFECTION
PLEASURES
MAGIC
INNER JOURNEY
BUT WHAT IF YOU WERE NEVER REALLY THAT INVESTED IN FEMININITY OR FERTILITY IN THE FIRST PLACE? WHAT ABOUT THOSE OF US WHOSE LIFE STAGES FOLLOW A DECIDEDLY QUEERER PATH?
THE STAGES OF LIFE: QUEER BLACK NERD EDITION
HOW'S THIS FOR A GAME? WE WATCH *ROSENCRANTZ & GUILDENSTERN ARE DEAD*, AND EACH TIME THEY QUOTE *HAMLET*, WE HAVE TO DRINK!
I CAN'T BELIEVE OUR HOUSE IS SCHEDULED TO CLOSE ON THE SAME DAY ALL MY BOOK EDITS ARE DUE!
I'M CURRENTLY WORKING ON A FEMINIST HISTORY OF THE ROLE OF THE COCKTAIL IN HARLEM RENAISSANCE LITERATURE.
ADVANCED PLACEMENT QUEER
MID CAREER QUEER
QUEER NERD EMERITUS

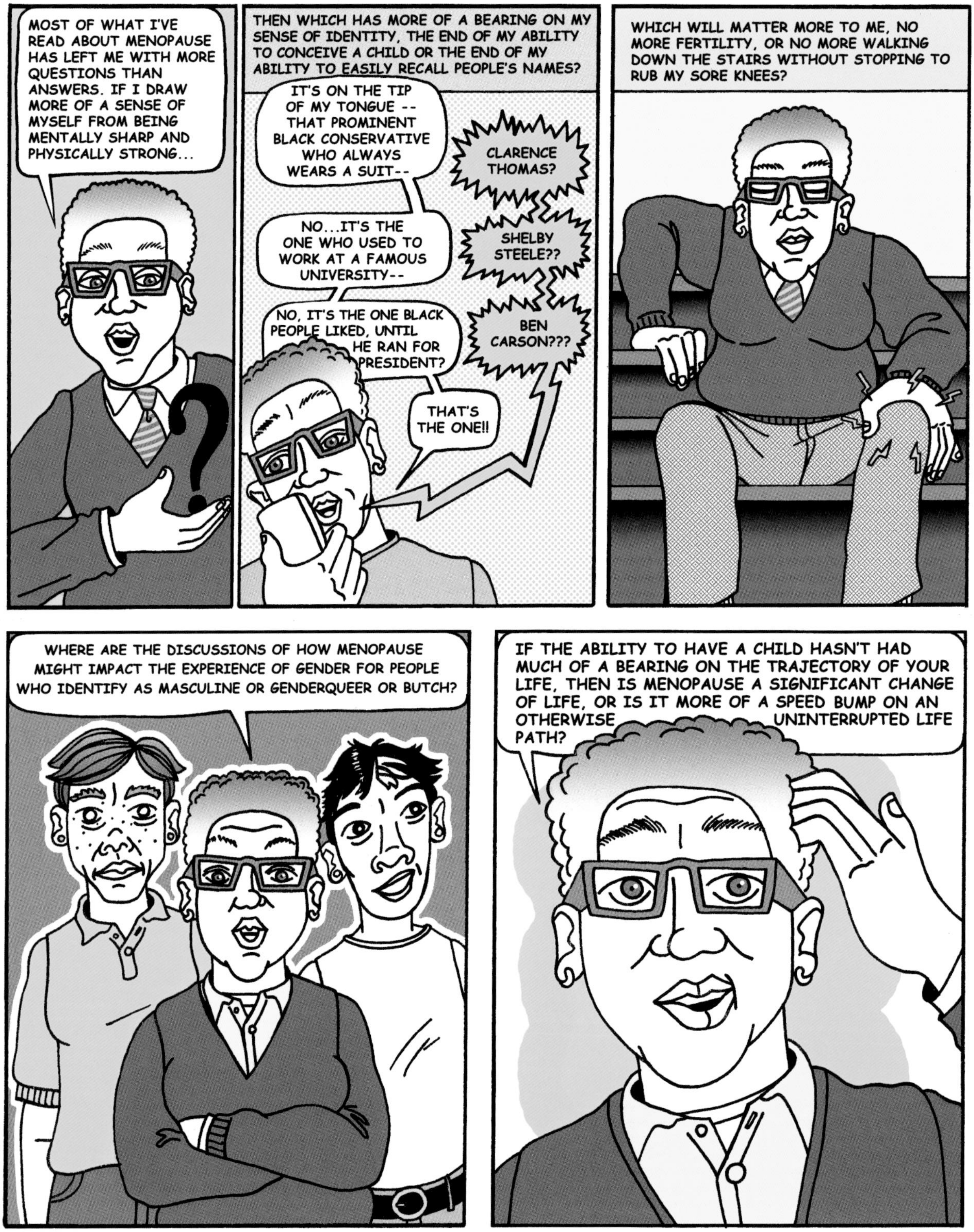
MOST OF WHAT I'VE READ ABOUT MENOPAUSE HAS LEFT ME WITH MORE QUESTIONS THAN ANSWERS. IF I DRAW MORE OF A SENSE OF MYSELF FROM BEING MENTALLY SHARP AND PHYSICALLY STRONG...
THEN WHICH HAS MORE OF A BEARING ON MY SENSE OF IDENTITY, THE END OF MY ABILITY TO CONCEIVE A CHILD OR THE END OF MY ABILITY TO EASILY RECALL PEOPLE'S NAMES?
IT'S ON THE TIP OF MY TONGUE -- THAT PROMINENT BLACK CONSERVATIVE WHO ALWAYS WEARS A SUIT--
CLARENCE THOMAS?
NO...IT'S THE ONE WHO USED TO WORK AT A FAMOUS UNIVERSITY--
SHELBY STEELE??
NO, IT'S THE ONE BLACK PEOPLE LIKED, UNTIL HE RAN FOR PRESIDENT?
BEN CARSON???
THAT'S THE ONE!!
WHICH WILL MATTER MORE TO ME, NO MORE FERTILITY, OR NO MORE WALKING DOWN THE STAIRS WITHOUT STOPPING TO RUB MY SORE KNEES?
WHERE ARE THE DISCUSSIONS OF HOW MENOPAUSE MIGHT IMPACT THE EXPERIENCE OF GENDER FOR PEOPLE WHO IDENTIFY AS MASCULINE OR GENDERQUEER OR BUTCH?
IF THE ABILITY TO HAVE A CHILD HASN'T HAD MUCH OF A BEARING ON THE TRAJECTORY OF YOUR LIFE, THEN IS MENOPAUSE A SIGNIFICANT CHANGE OF LIFE, OR IS IT MORE OF A SPEED BUMP ON AN OTHERWISE UNINTERRUPTED LIFE PATH?

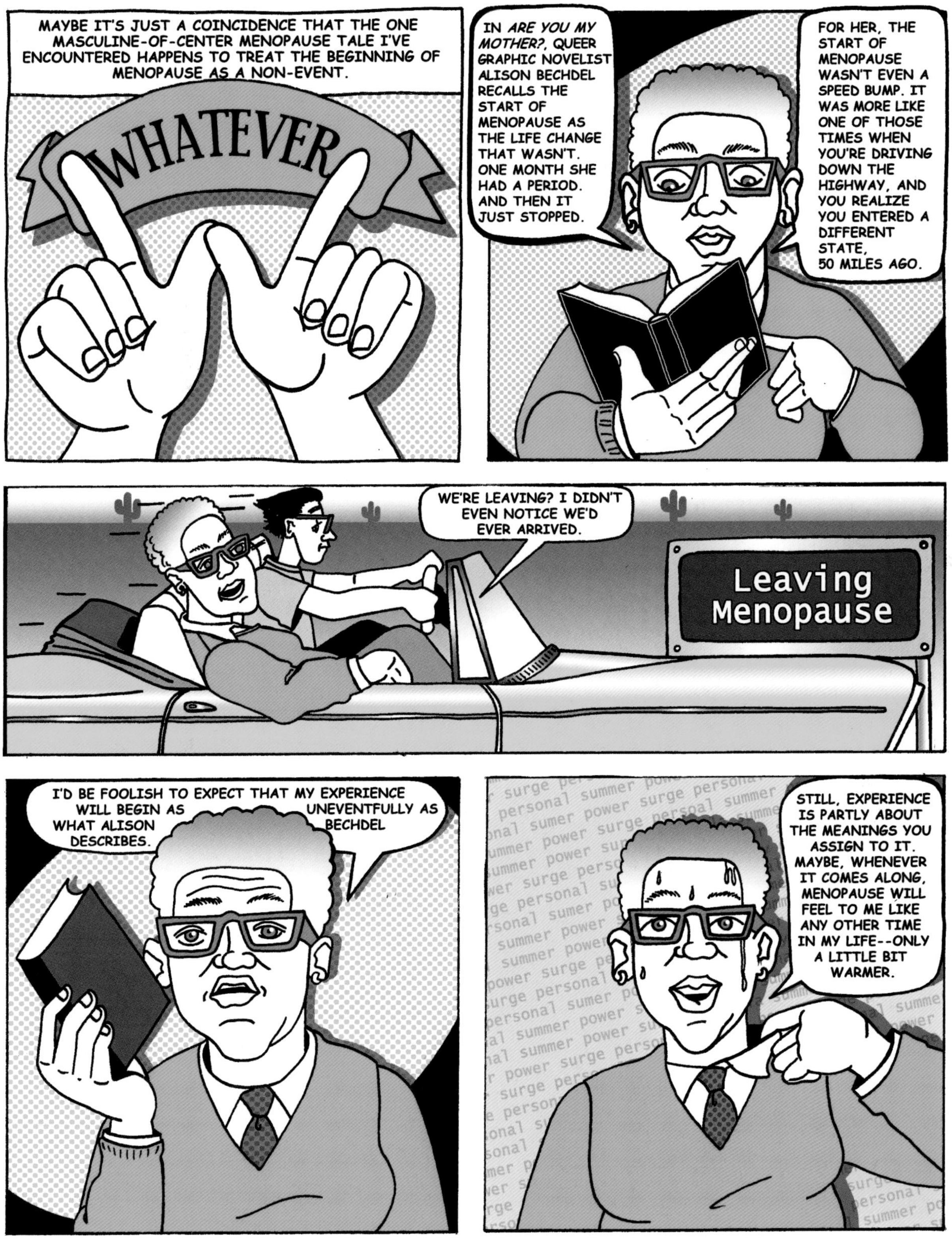
MAYBE IT'S JUST A COINCIDENCE THAT THE ONE MASCULINE-OF-CENTER MENOPAUSE TALE I'VE ENCOUNTERED HAPPENS TO TREAT THE BEGINNING OF MENOPAUSE AS A NON-EVENT.
WHATEVER
IN *ARE YOU MY MOTHER?*, QUEER GRAPHIC NOVELIST ALISON BECHDEL RECALLS THE START OF MENOPAUSE AS THE LIFE CHANGE THAT WASN'T. ONE MONTH SHE HAD A PERIOD. AND THEN IT JUST STOPPED.
FOR HER, THE START OF MENOPAUSE WASN'T EVEN A SPEED BUMP. IT WAS MORE LIKE ONE OF THOSE TIMES WHEN YOU'RE DRIVING DOWN THE HIGHWAY, AND YOU REALIZE YOU ENTERED A DIFFERENT STATE, 50 MILES AGO.
WE'RE LEAVING? I DIDN'T EVEN NOTICE WE'D EVER ARRIVED.
Leaving Menopause
I'D BE FOOLISH TO EXPECT THAT MY EXPERIENCE WILL BEGIN AS UNEVENTFULLY AS WHAT ALISON BECHDEL DESCRIBES.
STILL, EXPERIENCE IS PARTLY ABOUT THE MEANINGS YOU ASSIGN TO IT. MAYBE, WHENEVER IT COMES ALONG, MENOPAUSE WILL FEEL TO ME LIKE ANY OTHER TIME IN MY LIFE--ONLY A LITTLE BIT WARMER.

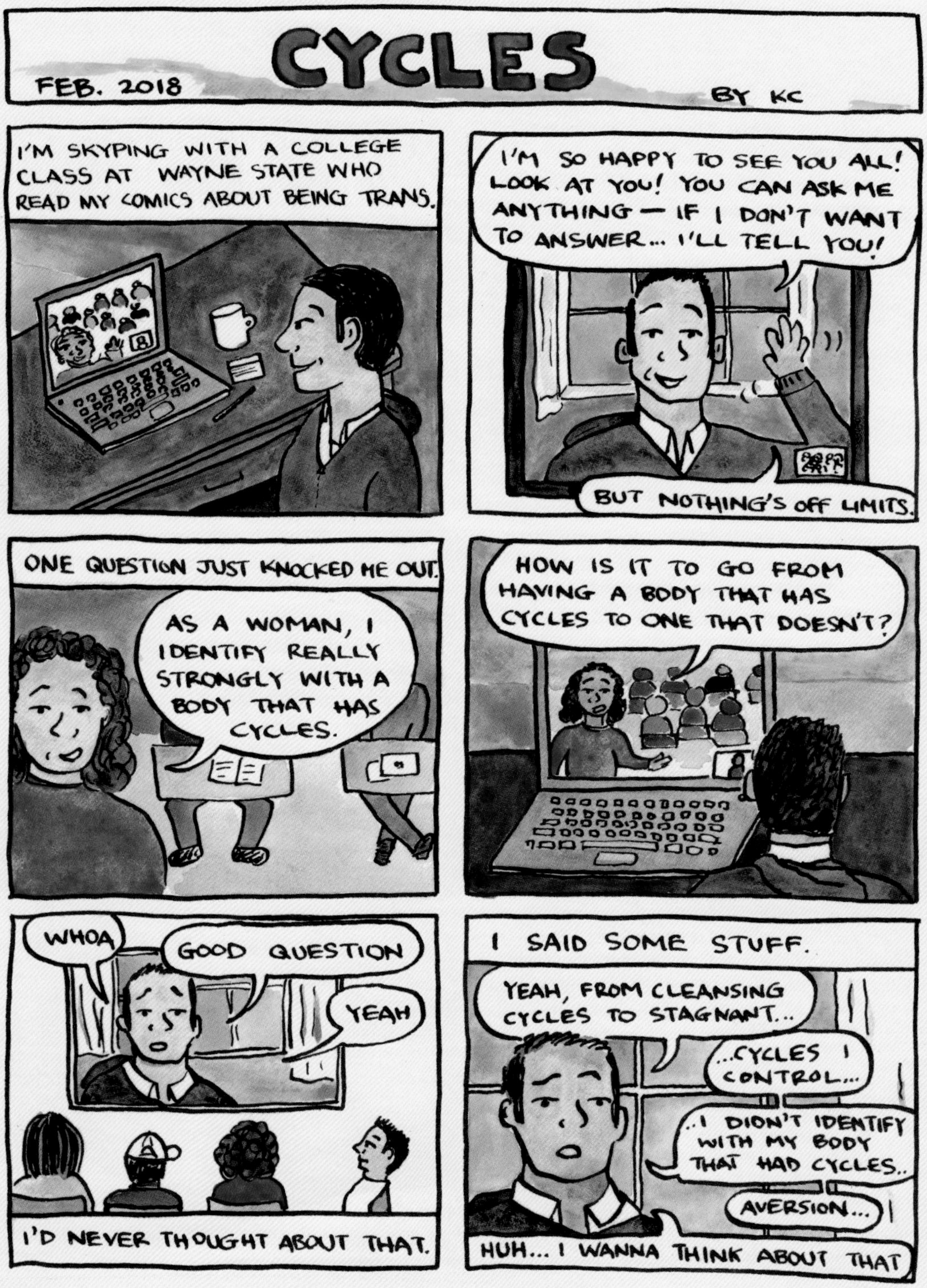
CYCLES
FEB. 2018
BY KC
I'M SKYPING WITH A COLLEGE CLASS AT WAYNE STATE WHO READ MY COMICS ABOUT BEING TRANS.
I'M SO HAPPY TO SEE YOU ALL! LOOK AT YOU! YOU CAN ASK ME ANYTHING — IF I DON'T WANT TO ANSWER... I'LL TELL YOU!
BUT NOTHING'S OFF LIMITS.
ONE QUESTION JUST KNOCKED ME OUT.
AS A WOMAN, I IDENTIFY REALLY STRONGLY WITH A BODY THAT HAS CYCLES.
HOW IS IT TO GO FROM HAVING A BODY THAT HAS CYCLES TO ONE THAT DOESN'T?
WHOA
GOOD QUESTION
YEAH
I'D NEVER THOUGHT ABOUT THAT.
I SAID SOME STUFF.
YEAH, FROM CLEANSING CYCLES TO STAGNANT...
...CYCLES I CONTROL...
...I DIDN'T IDENTIFY WITH MY BODY THAT HAD CYCLES..
AVERSION...
HUH... I WANNA THINK ABOUT THAT

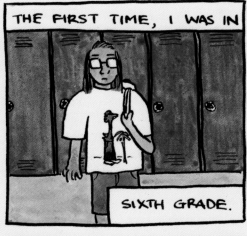

THE FIRST TIME, I WAS IN

SIXTH GRADE.

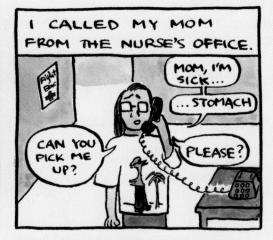

I CALLED MY MOM FROM THE NURSE'S OFFICE.

MOM, I'M SICK...

...STOMACH

CAN YOU PICK ME UP?

PLEASE?

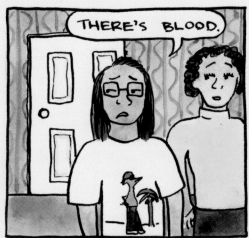

THERE'S BLOOD.

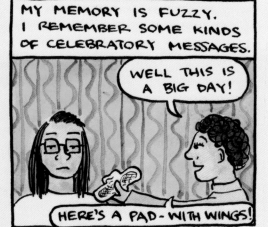

MY MEMORY IS FUZZY. I REMEMBER SOME KINDS OF CELEBRATORY MESSAGES.

WELL THIS IS A BIG DAY!

HERE'S A PAD - WITH WINGS!

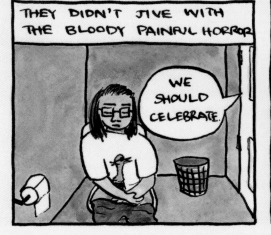

THEY DIDN'T JIVE WITH THE BLOODY PAINFUL HORROR

WE SHOULD CELEBRATE.

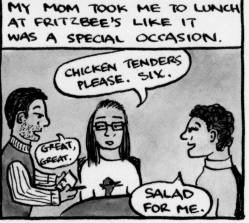

MY MOM TOOK ME TO LUNCH AT FRITZBEE'S LIKE IT WAS A SPECIAL OCCASION.

CHICKEN TENDERS PLEASE. SIX.

GREAT, GREAT.

SALAD FOR ME.

I REMEMBER THAT NIGHT AT DINNER MY DAD SAID SOMETHING.

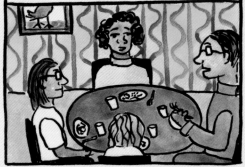

YOUR MOM TELLS ME YOU'RE A WOMAN NOW. THAT'S A BIG DEAL.

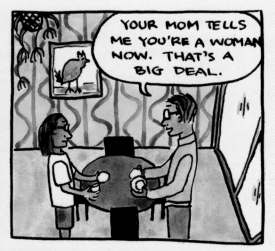

FROM THEN ON, MY FAVORITE DAY OF THE MONTH WAS THE FIRST DAY AFTER MY PERIOD.

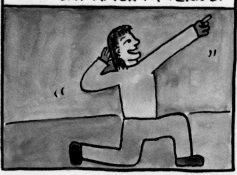

THEN EVERY DAY AFTER WAS A DESCENT LIKE THE ONE INTO WINTER—DREAD, DARKNESS.

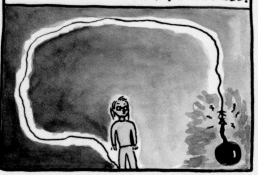

I DON'T KNOW HOW TO DESCRIBE WHAT IT'S LIKE TO BE OVERTAKEN BY THE PHYSICALITY OF BEING A WOMAN

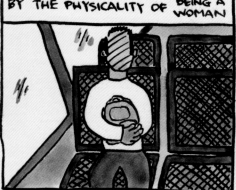

WHEN THAT'S NOT WHO YOU ARE.

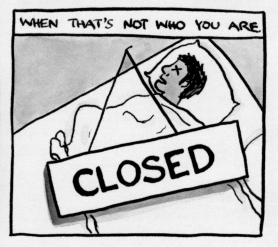

CLOSED

3

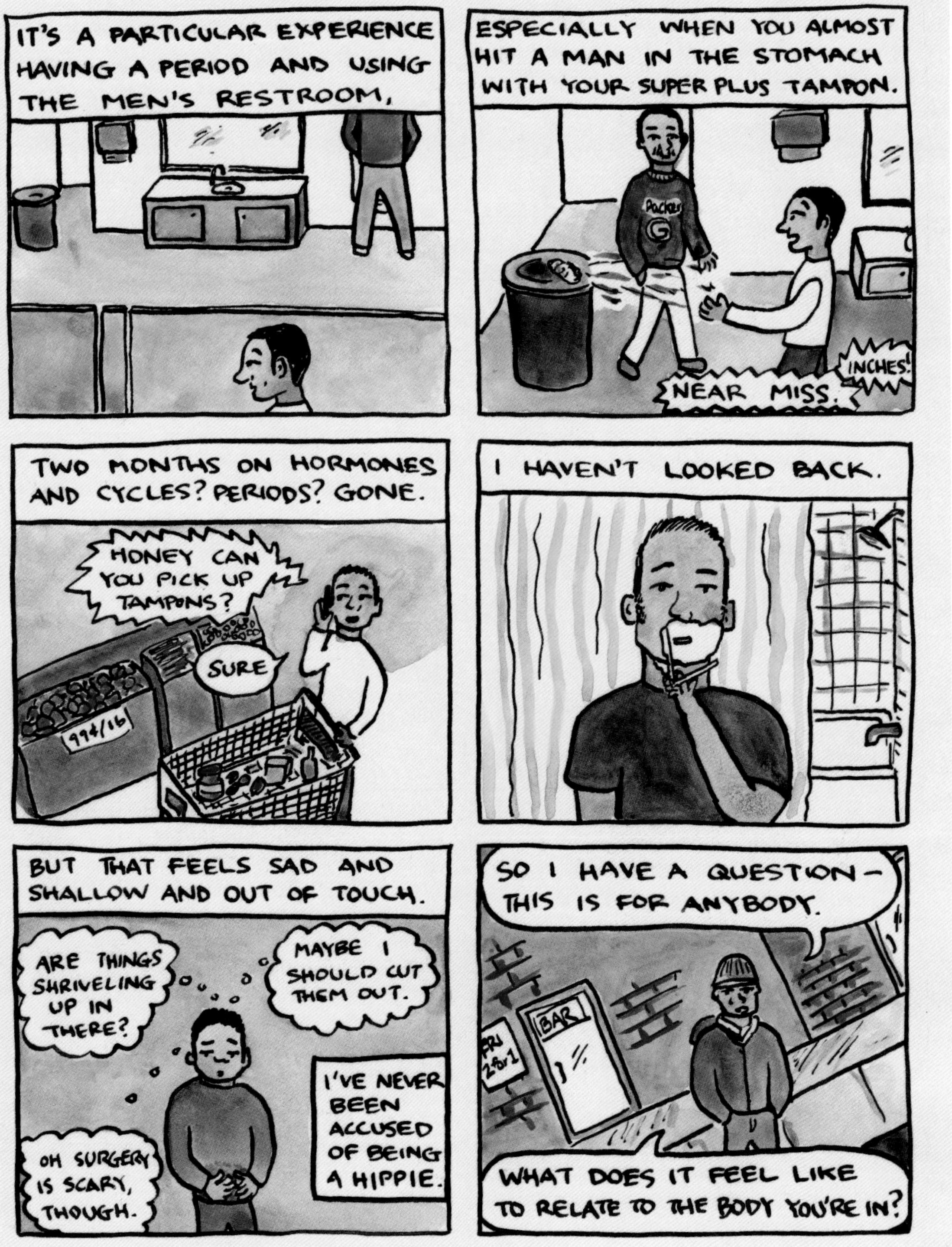
IT'S A PARTICULAR EXPERIENCE HAVING A PERIOD AND USING THE MEN'S RESTROOM,
ESPECIALLY WHEN YOU ALMOST HIT A MAN IN THE STOMACH WITH YOUR SUPER PLUS TAMPON.
Packers
G
NEAR MISS.
INCHES!
TWO MONTHS ON HORMONES AND CYCLES? PERIODS? GONE.
HONEY CAN YOU PICK UP TAMPONS?
SURE
99¢/lb
I HAVEN'T LOOKED BACK.
BUT THAT FEELS SAD AND SHALLOW AND OUT OF TOUCH.
ARE THINGS SHRIVELING UP IN THERE?
MAYBE I SHOULD CUT THEM OUT.
OH SURGERY IS SCARY, THOUGH.
I'VE NEVER BEEN ACCUSED OF BEING A HIPPIE.
SO I HAVE A QUESTION— THIS IS FOR ANYBODY.
FRI 2 for 1
BAR
WHAT DOES IT FEEL LIKE TO RELATE TO THE BODY YOU'RE IN?
4

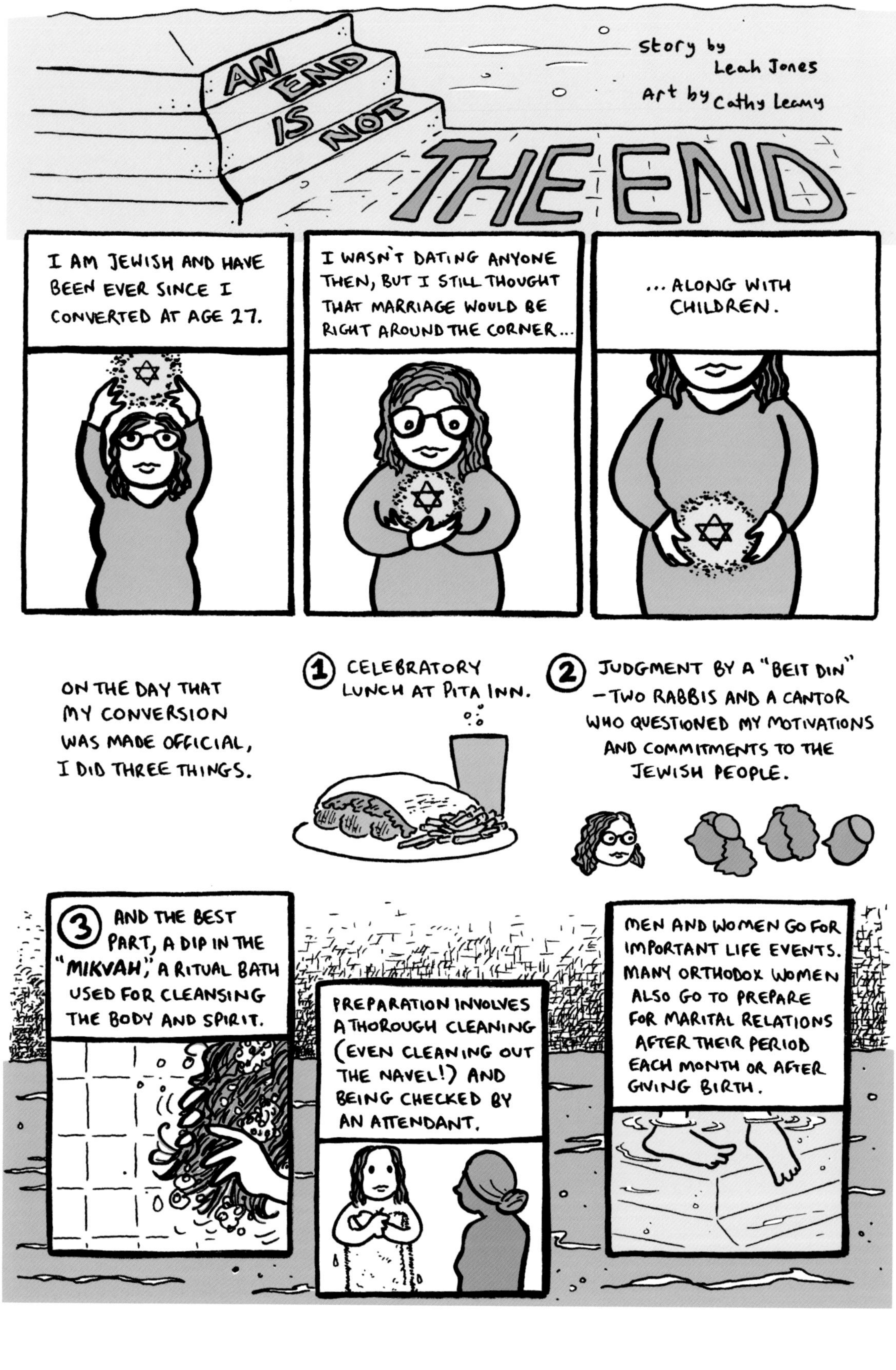
AN END IS NOT THE END
story by Leah Jones
Art by Cathy Leamy
I AM JEWISH AND HAVE BEEN EVER SINCE I CONVERTED AT AGE 27.
I WASN'T DATING ANYONE THEN, BUT I STILL THOUGHT THAT MARRIAGE WOULD BE RIGHT AROUND THE CORNER...
...ALONG WITH CHILDREN.
ON THE DAY THAT MY CONVERSION WAS MADE OFFICIAL, I DID THREE THINGS.
1 CELEBRATORY LUNCH AT PITA INN.
2 JUDGMENT BY A "BEIT DIN" —TWO RABBIS AND A CANTOR WHO QUESTIONED MY MOTIVATIONS AND COMMITMENTS TO THE JEWISH PEOPLE.
3 AND THE BEST PART, A DIP IN THE "MIKVAH," A RITUAL BATH USED FOR CLEANSING THE BODY AND SPIRIT.
PREPARATION INVOLVES A THOROUGH CLEANING (EVEN CLEANING OUT THE NAVEL!) AND BEING CHECKED BY AN ATTENDANT.
MEN AND WOMEN GO FOR IMPORTANT LIFE EVENTS. MANY ORTHODOX WOMEN ALSO GO TO PREPARE FOR MARITAL RELATIONS AFTER THEIR PERIOD EACH MONTH OR AFTER GIVING BIRTH.

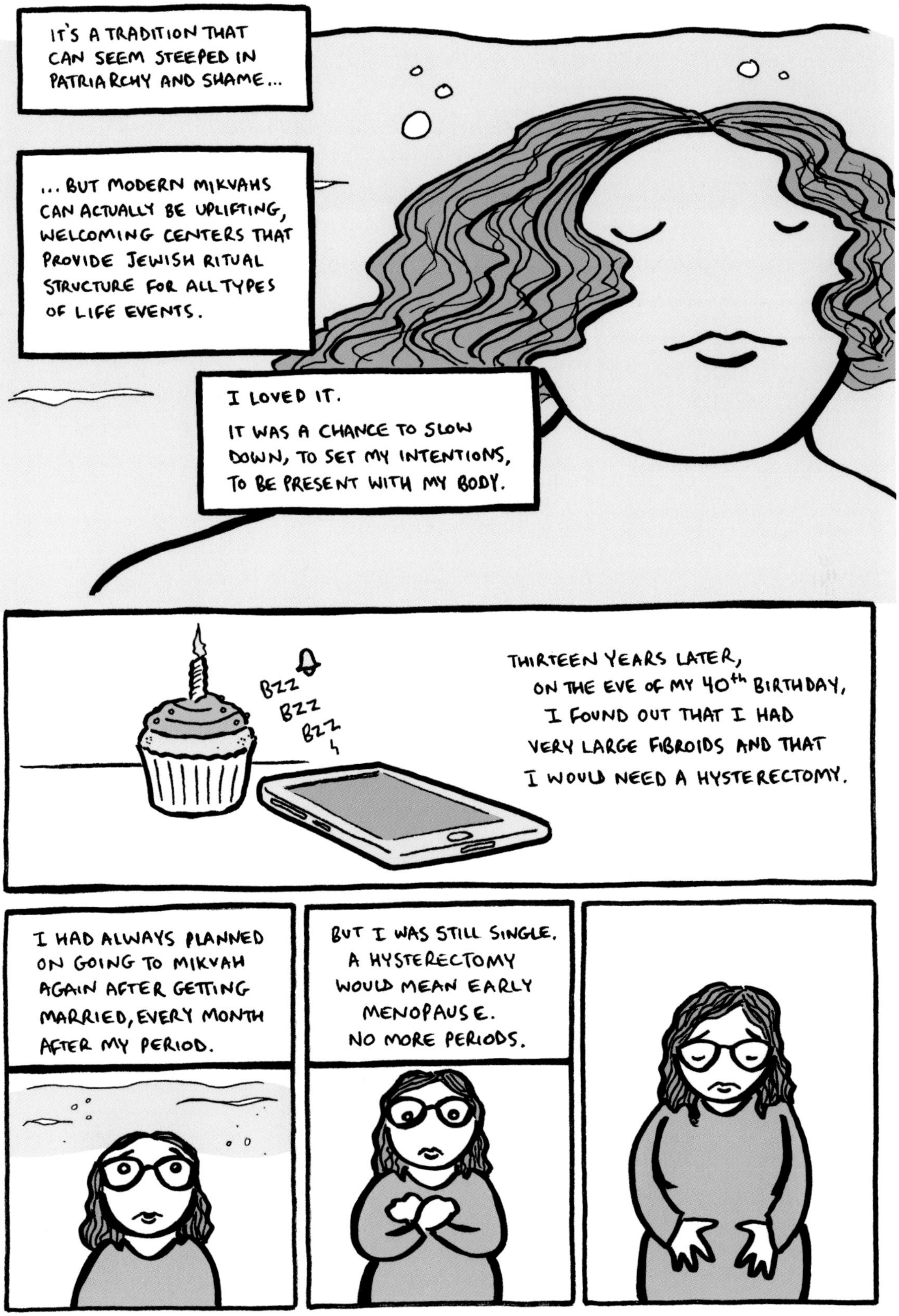
IT'S A TRADITION THAT CAN SEEM STEEPED IN PATRIARCHY AND SHAME...
...BUT MODERN MIKVAHS CAN ACTUALLY BE UPLIFTING, WELCOMING CENTERS THAT PROVIDE JEWISH RITUAL STRUCTURE FOR ALL TYPES OF LIFE EVENTS.
I LOVED IT.
IT WAS A CHANCE TO SLOW DOWN, TO SET MY INTENTIONS, TO BE PRESENT WITH MY BODY.
BZZ BZZ BZZ
THIRTEEN YEARS LATER, ON THE EVE OF MY 40th BIRTHDAY, I FOUND OUT THAT I HAD VERY LARGE FIBROIDS AND THAT I WOULD NEED A HYSTERECTOMY.
I HAD ALWAYS PLANNED ON GOING TO MIKVAH AGAIN AFTER GETTING MARRIED, EVERY MONTH AFTER MY PERIOD.
BUT I WAS STILL SINGLE. A HYSTERECTOMY WOULD MEAN EARLY MENOPAUSE. NO MORE PERIODS.

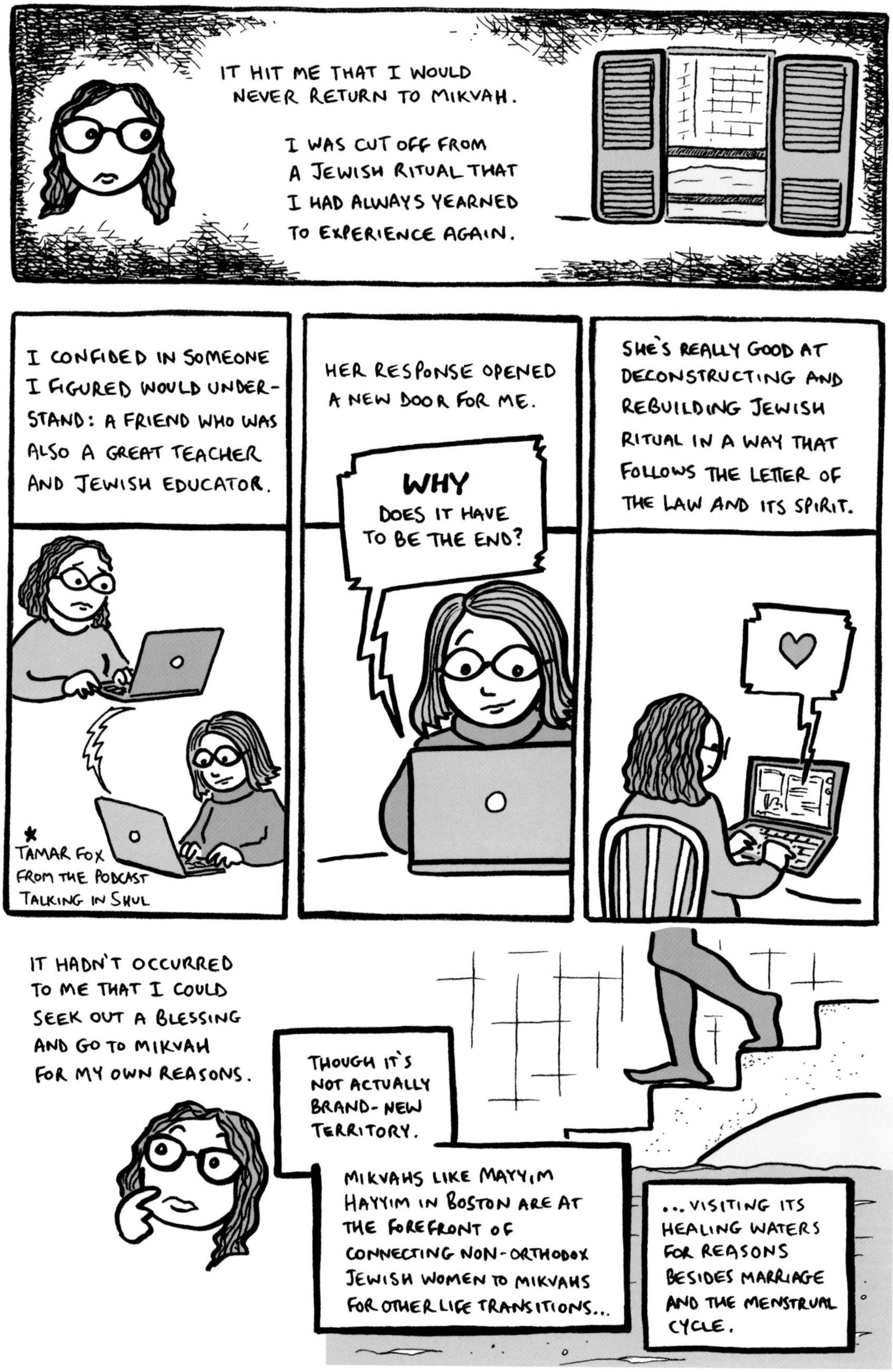
IT HIT ME THAT I WOULD NEVER RETURN TO MIKVAH.
I WAS CUT OFF FROM A JEWISH RITUAL THAT I HAD ALWAYS YEARNED TO EXPERIENCE AGAIN.
I CONFIDED IN SOMEONE I FIGURED WOULD UNDER-STAND: A FRIEND WHO WAS ALSO A GREAT TEACHER AND JEWISH EDUCATOR.
* TAMAR FOX FROM THE PODCAST TALKING IN SHUL
HER RESPONSE OPENED A NEW DOOR FOR ME.
WHY DOES IT HAVE TO BE THE END?
SHE'S REALLY GOOD AT DECONSTRUCTING AND REBUILDING JEWISH RITUAL IN A WAY THAT FOLLOWS THE LETTER OF THE LAW AND ITS SPIRIT.
IT HADN'T OCCURRED TO ME THAT I COULD SEEK OUT A BLESSING AND GO TO MIKVAH FOR MY OWN REASONS.
THOUGH IT'S NOT ACTUALLY BRAND-NEW TERRITORY.
MIKVAHS LIKE MAYYIM HAYYIM IN BOSTON ARE AT THE FOREFRONT OF CONNECTING NON-ORTHODOX JEWISH WOMEN TO MIKVAHS FOR OTHER LIFE TRANSITIONS...
...VISITING ITS HEALING WATERS FOR REASONS BESIDES MARRIAGE AND THE MENSTRUAL CYCLE.

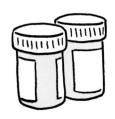
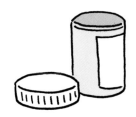

THIS TIME, PREPARING FOR MIKVAH INVOLVED SOME DIFFERENT PLANNING.

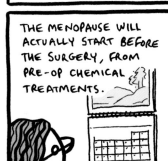

THE MENOPAUSE WILL ACTUALLY START BEFORE THE SURGERY, FROM PRE-OP CHEMICAL TREATMENTS.

TIME PRESSURE TO FIGURE THINGS OUT BEFORE THAT TREATMENT DAY!

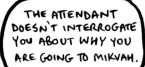

THE ATTENDANT DOESN'T INTERROGATE YOU ABOUT WHY YOU ARE GOING TO MIKVAH.

YOU'LL BE OK GOING FOR YOUR OWN SPECIFIC REASONS.

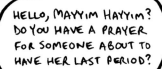

HELLO, MAYYIM HAYYIM? DO YOU HAVE A PRAYER FOR SOMEONE ABOUT TO HAVE HER LAST PERIOD?

UH, MOST WOMEN DON'T KNOW WHEN THAT IS, SO...

...NO?

(THEY SENT A PRAYER OF HEALING INSTEAD.)

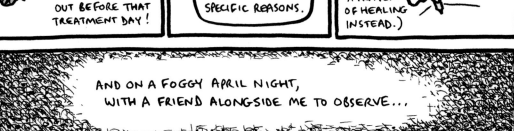

AND ON A FOGGY APRIL NIGHT, WITH A FRIEND ALONGSIDE ME TO OBSERVE...

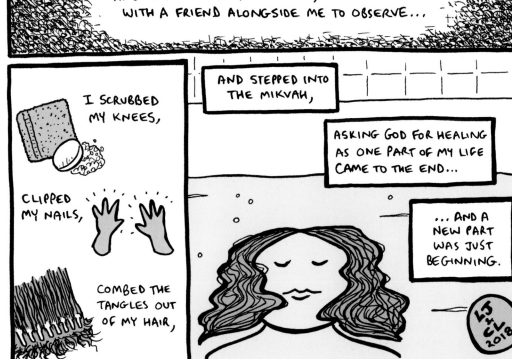

I SCRUBBED MY KNEES,

CLIPPED MY NAILS,

COMBED THE TANGLES OUT OF MY HAIR,

AND STEPPED INTO THE MIKVAH,

ASKING GOD FOR HEALING AS ONE PART OF MY LIFE CAME TO THE END...

...AND A NEW PART WAS JUST BEGINNING.

LJ & CL 2018

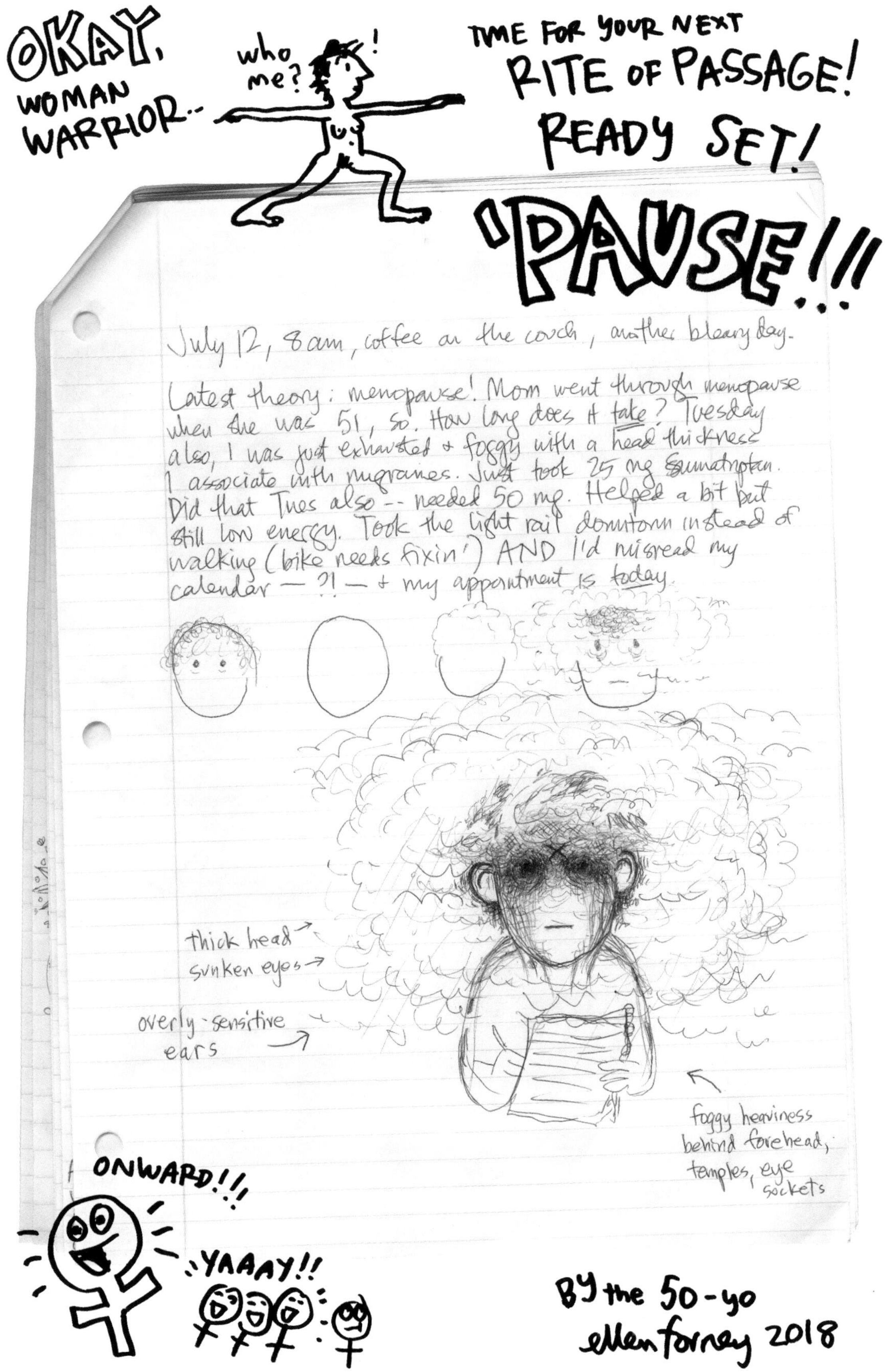

OKAY, WOMAN WARRIOR..
who me?!
TIME FOR YOUR NEXT RITE OF PASSAGE!
READY SET!
'PAUSE!!!
July 12, 8 am, coffee on the couch, another bleary day.
Latest theory: menopause! Mom went through menopause when she was 51, so. How long does it take? Tuesday also, I was just exhausted & foggy with a head thickness I associate with migraines. Just took 25 mg Sumatriptan. Did that Tues also -- needed 50 mg. Helped a bit but still low energy. Took the light rail downtown instead of walking (bike needs fixin') AND I'd misread my calendar — ?! — & my appointment is today.
thick head
sunken eyes
overly-sensitive ears
foggy heaviness behind forehead, temples, eye sockets
ONWARD!!!
YAAAY!!
BY the 50-yo ellen forney 2018

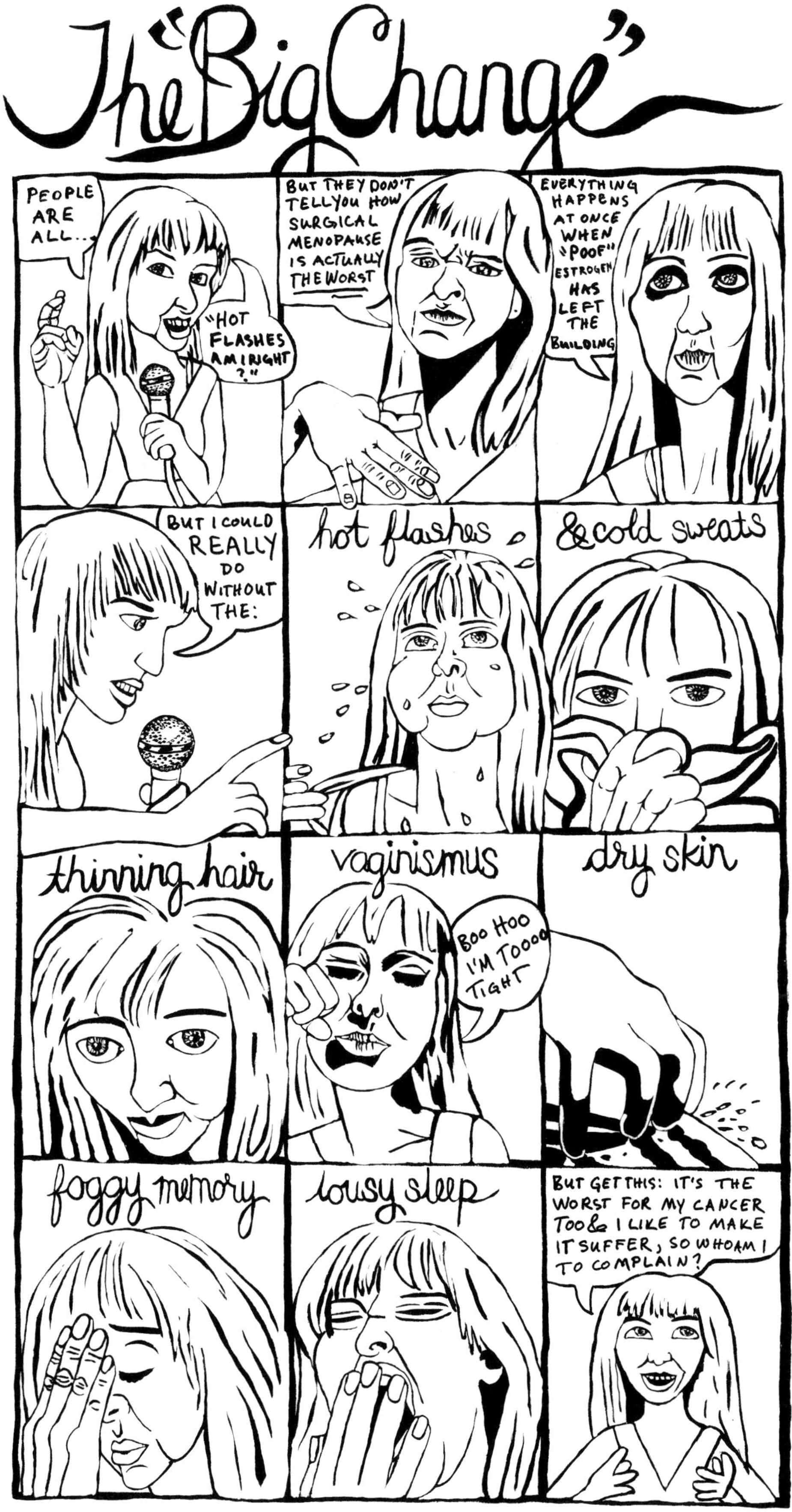
"The Big Change"
PEOPLE ARE ALL...
"HOT FLASHES AMIRIGHT?"
BUT THEY DON'T TELL YOU HOW SURGICAL MENOPAUSE IS ACTUALLY THE WORST
EVERYTHING HAPPENS AT ONCE WHEN "POOF" ESTROGEN HAS LEFT THE BUILDING
BUT I COULD REALLY DO WITHOUT THE:
hot flashes
& cold sweats
thinning hair
vaginismus
BOO HOO I'M TOOOO TIGHT
dry skin
foggy memory
lousy sleep
BUT GET THIS: IT'S THE WORST FOR MY CANCER TOO & I LIKE TO MAKE IT SUFFER, SO WHO AM I TO COMPLAIN?

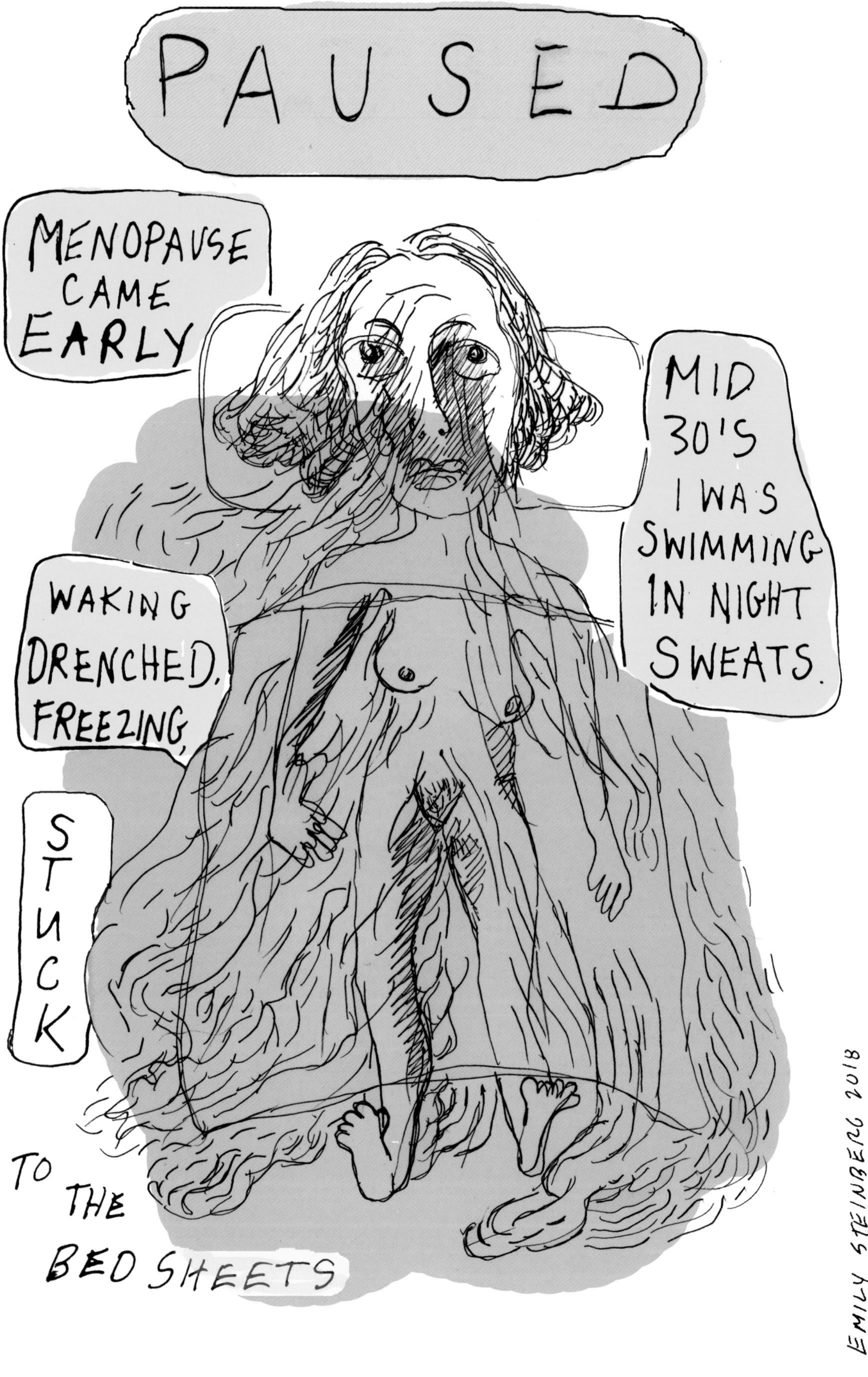
PAUSED
MENOPAUSE CAME EARLY
MID 30'S I WAS SWIMMING IN NIGHT SWEATS.
WAKING DRENCHED, FREEZING,
STUCK
TO THE BED SHEETS
EMILY STEINBERG 2018

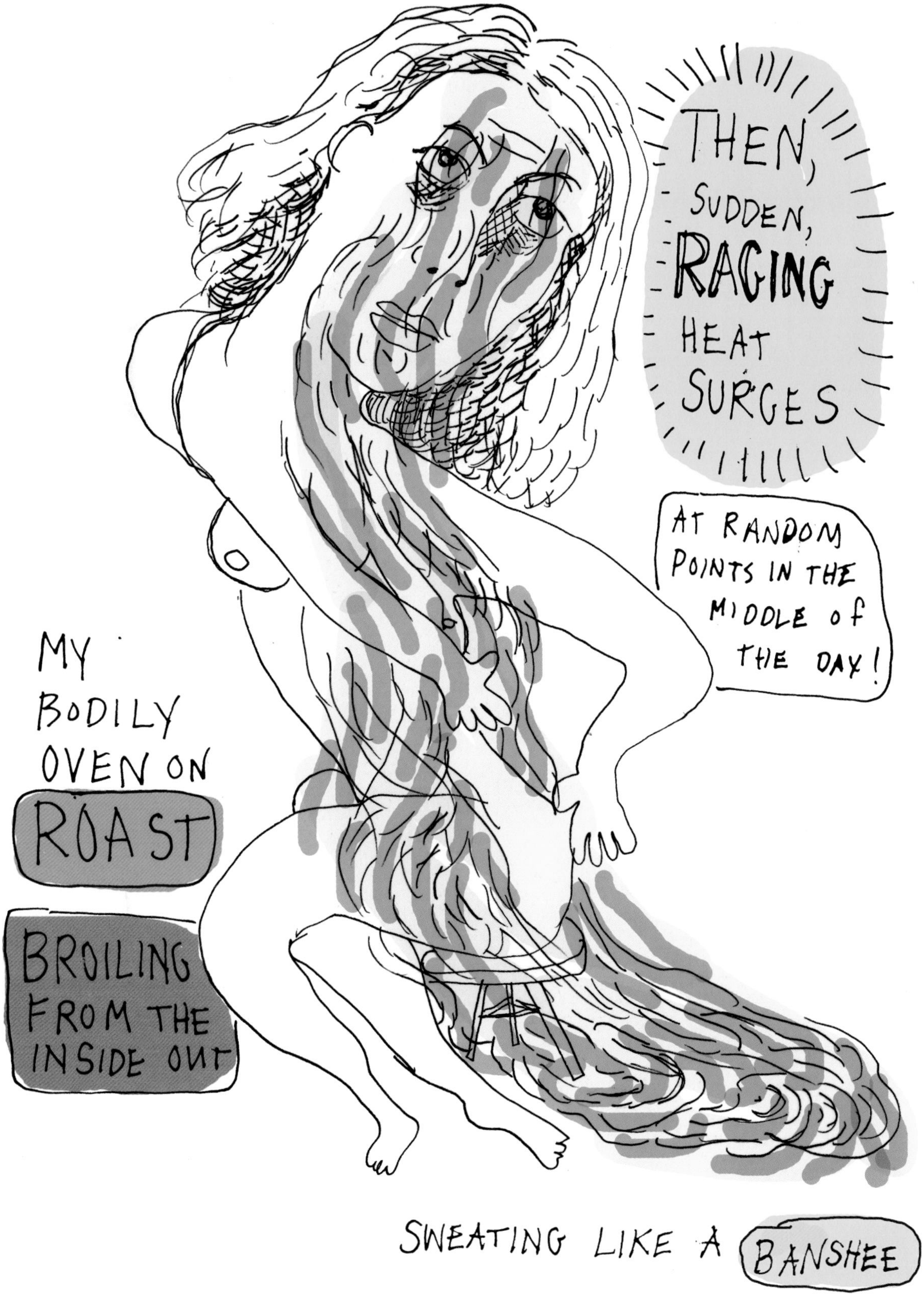
THEN, SUDDEN, RAGING HEAT SURGES
AT RANDOM POINTS IN THE MIDDLE OF THE DAY!
MY BODILY OVEN ON
ROAST
BROILING FROM THE INSIDE OUT
SWEATING LIKE A BANSHEE

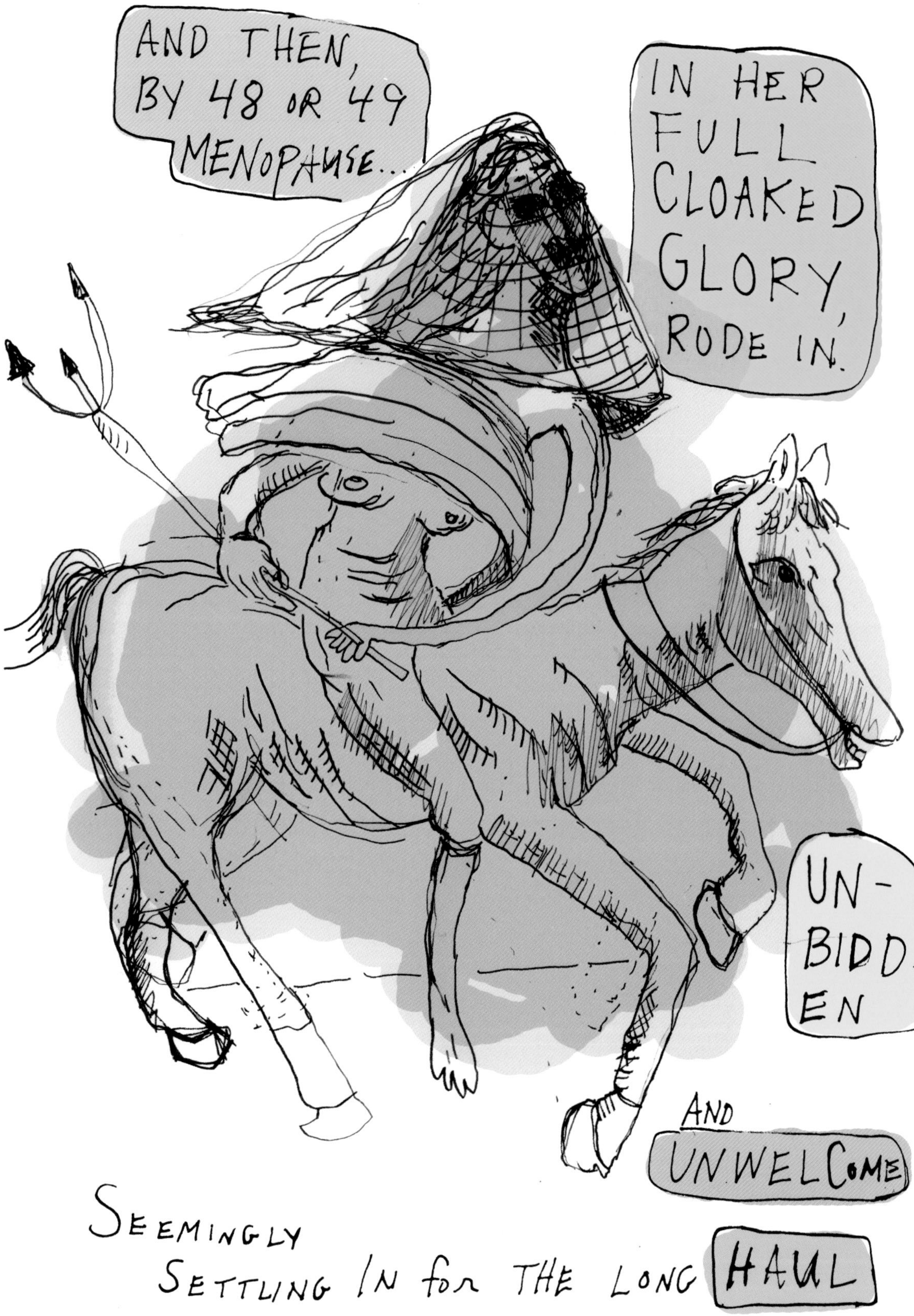
AND THEN, BY 48 OR 49 MENOPAUSE...
IN HER FULL CLOAKED GLORY, RODE IN.
UN-BIDD-EN
AND UNWELCOME
SEEMINGLY SETTLING IN for THE LONG HAUL

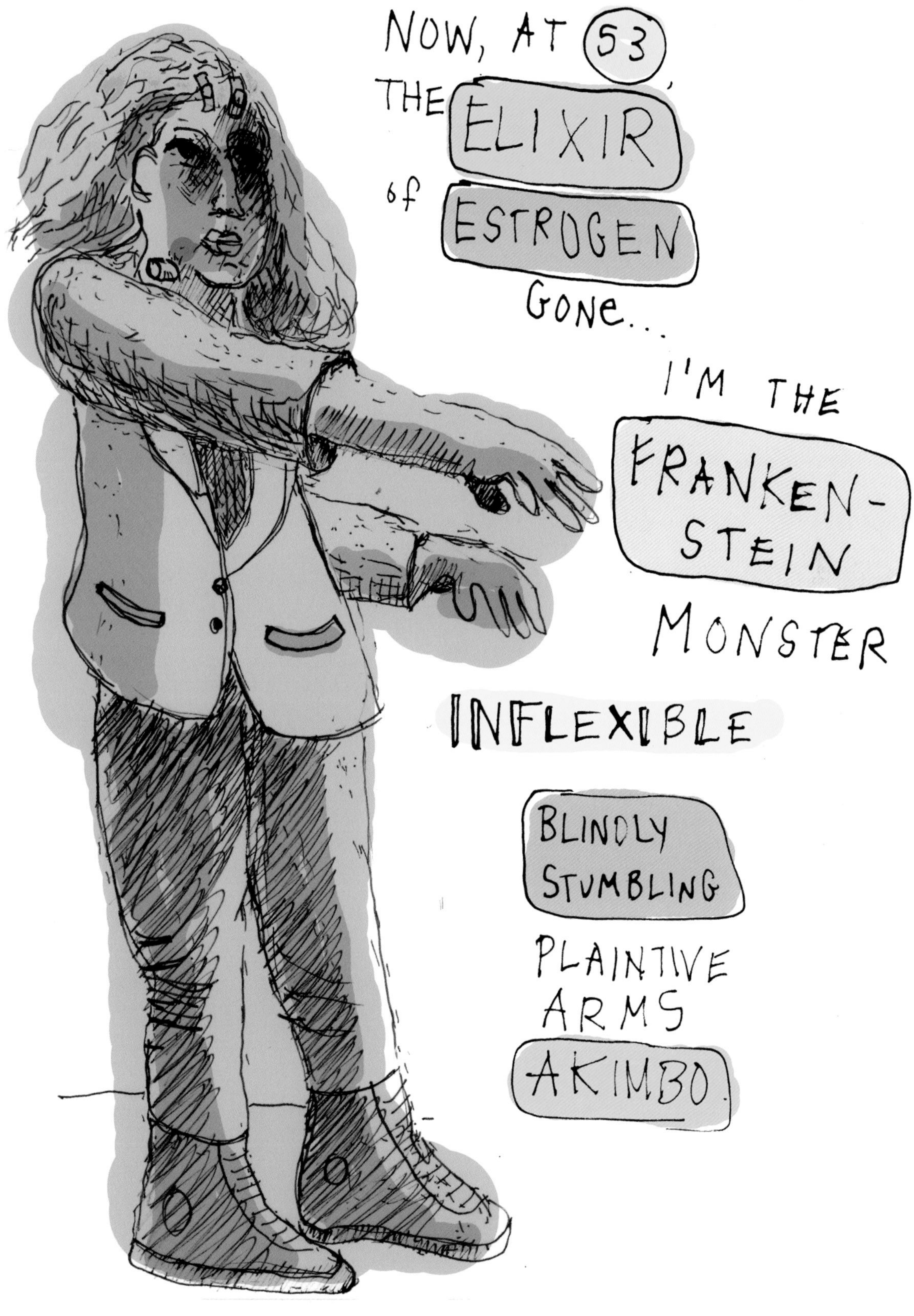
NOW, AT 53,
THE ELIXIR
of ESTROGEN
GONE...
I'M THE
FRANKEN-
STEIN
MONSTER
INFLEXIBLE
BLINDLY
STUMBLING
PLAINTIVE
ARMS
AKIMBO

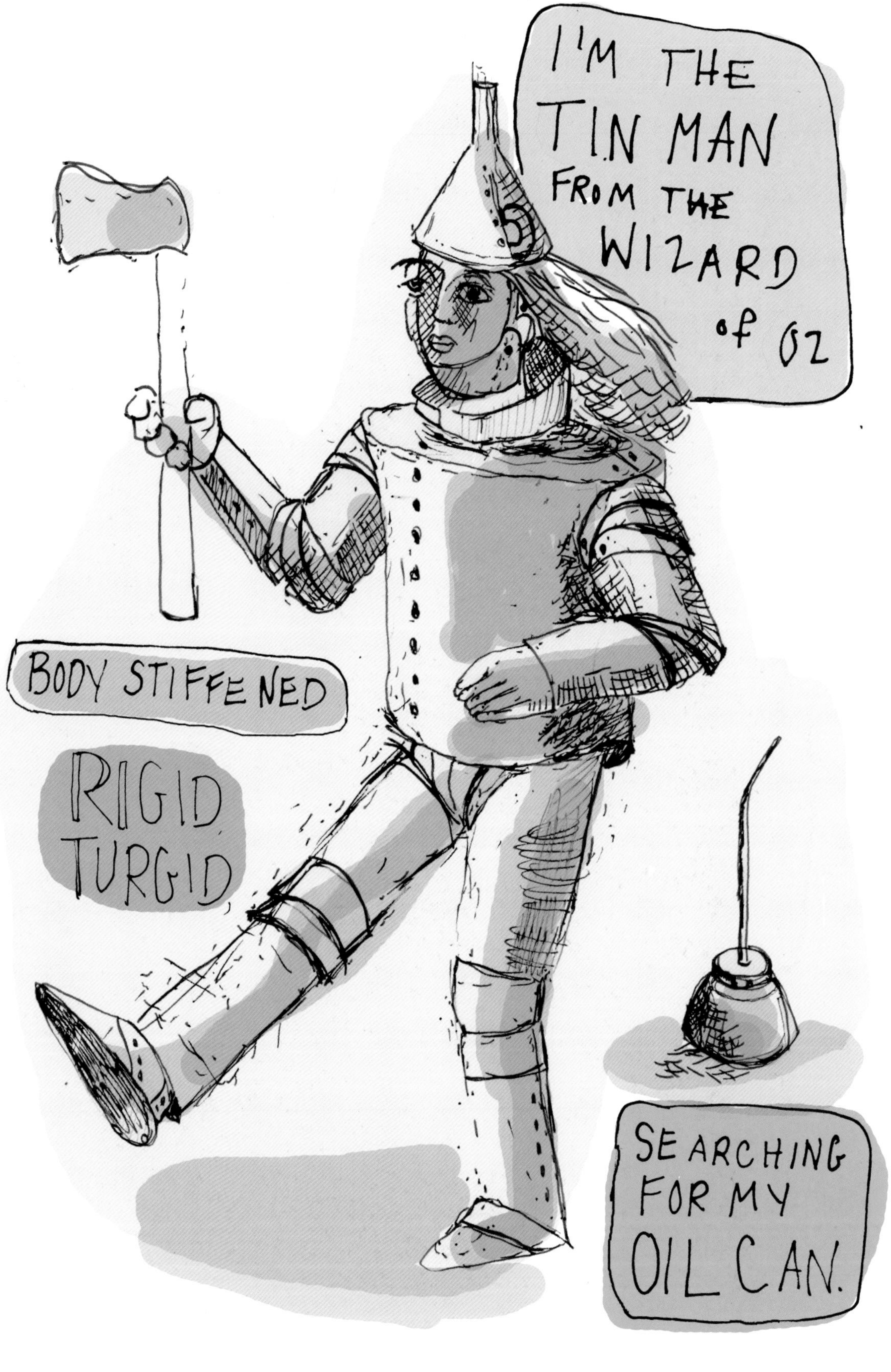
I'M THE TIN MAN FROM THE WIZARD of OZ
BODY STIFFENED
RIGID TURGID
SEARCHING FOR MY OIL CAN.

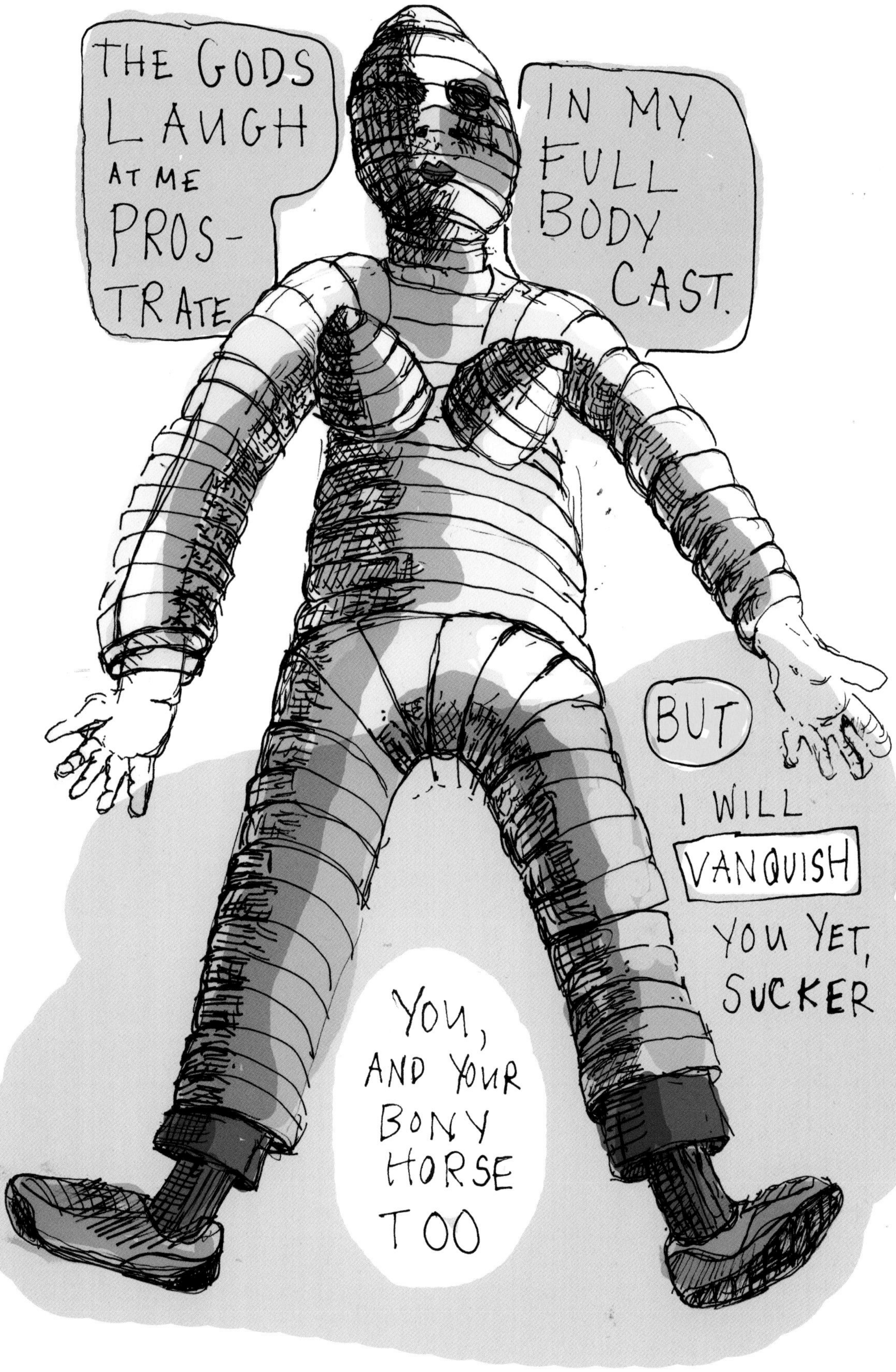
THE GODS LAUGH AT ME PROS-TRATE
IN MY FULL BODY CAST.
BUT
I WILL VANQUISH YOU YET, SUCKER
YOU, AND YOUR BONY HORSE TOO

KIMIKO DOES MENOPAUSE*

BY KIMIKO TOBIMATSU & KEET GENIZA

After getting estrogen-positive breast cancer at 25, I was put into menopause to prevent recurrence. I'm still working out how to explain what it's like.

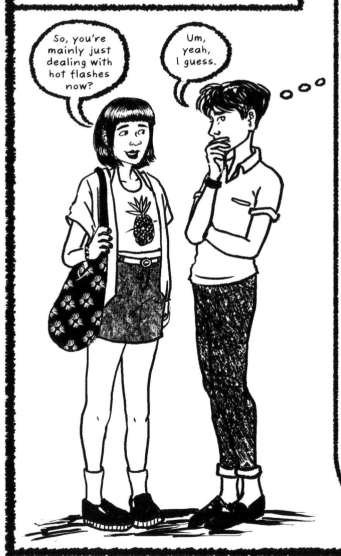

So, you're mainly just dealing with hot flashes now?

Um, yeah, I guess.

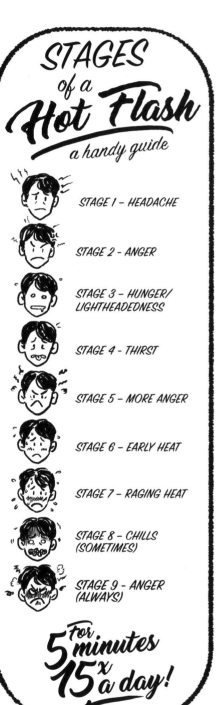

STAGES of a Hot Flash

a handy guide

STAGE 1 – HEADACHE

STAGE 2 – ANGER

STAGE 3 – HUNGER/LIGHTHEADEDNESS

STAGE 4 – THIRST

STAGE 5 – MORE ANGER

STAGE 6 – EARLY HEAT

STAGE 7 – RAGING HEAT

STAGE 8 – CHILLS (SOMETIMES)

STAGE 9 – ANGER (ALWAYS)

For 5 minutes 15x a day!

*EXCERPT FROM UPCOMING GRAPHIC MEMOIR, KIMIKO DOES CANCER

SURGICAL MENOPAUSE – IN TEN POSTURES

SUSAN MERRILL SQUIER
SHELLEY L. WALL

ONE: POWER POSE

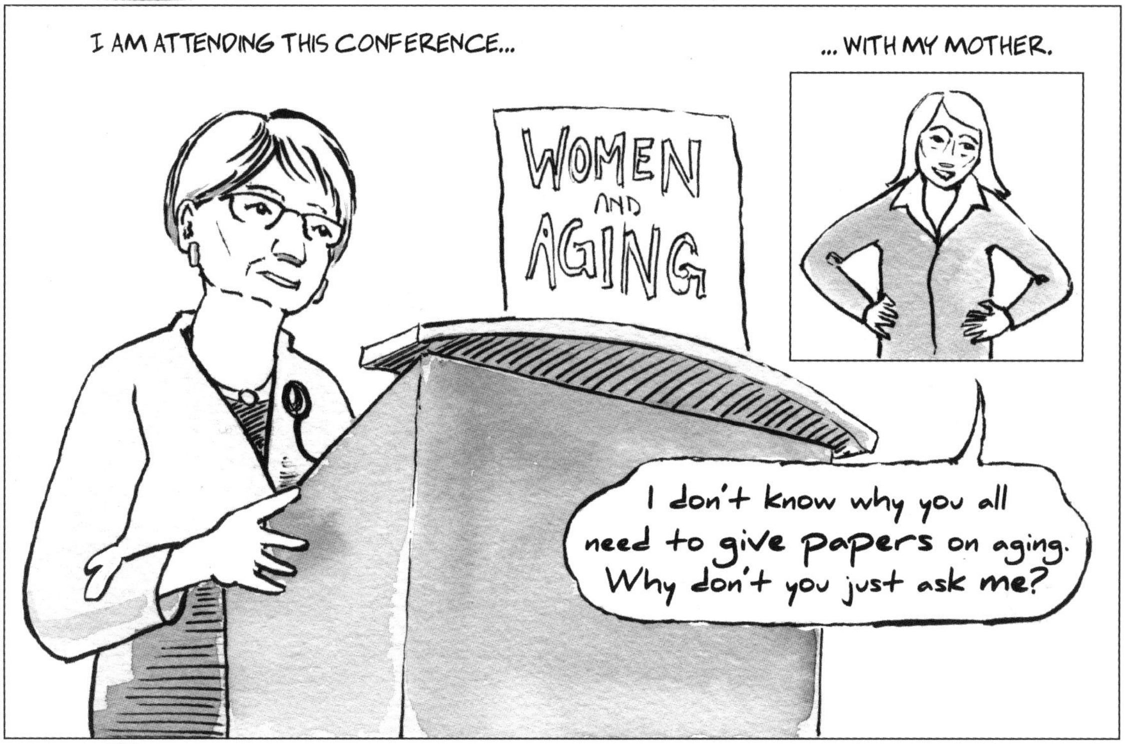
I AM ATTENDING THIS CONFERENCE...
... WITH MY MOTHER.
WOMEN AND AGING
I don't know why you all need to give papers on aging. Why don't you just ask me?

TWO: COMMA

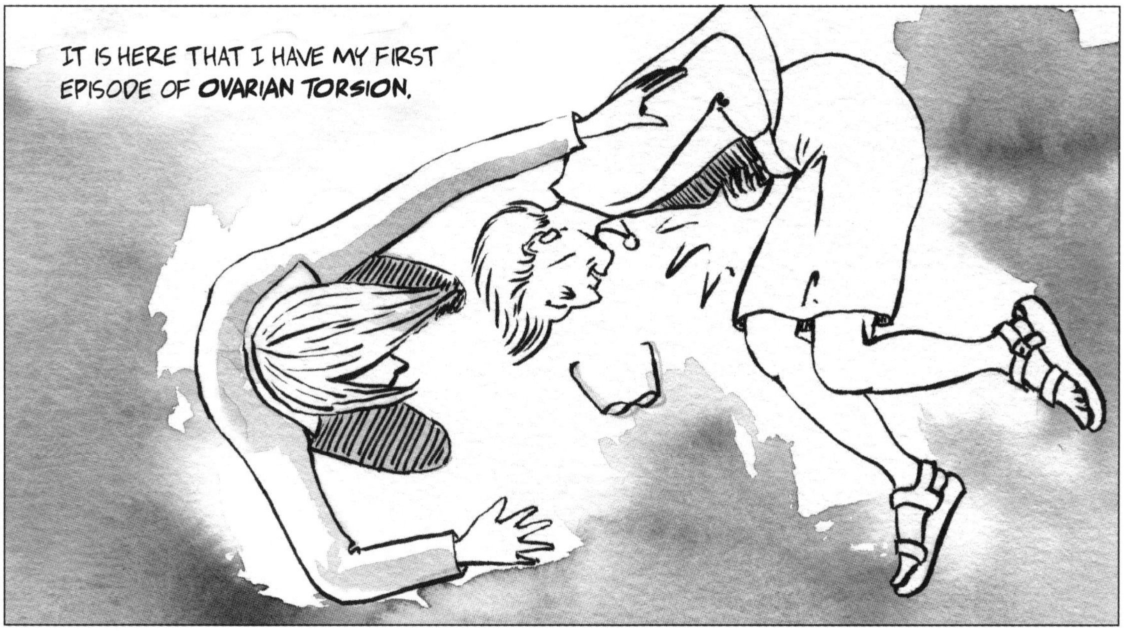
IT IS HERE THAT I HAVE MY FIRST EPISODE OF **OVARIAN TORSION**.

THREE: STRIPPING

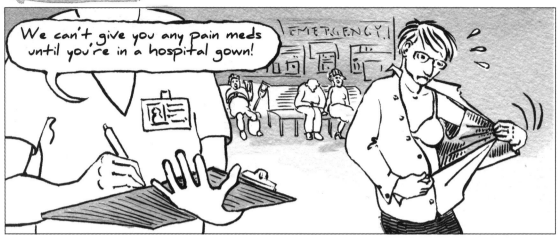

We can't give you any pain meds until you're in a hospital gown!

EMERGENCY.

FOUR: SUPINE, WITH PROD

I HAVE A TRANSVAGINAL ULTRASOUND...

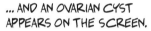... AND AN OVARIAN CYST APPEARS ON THE SCREEN.

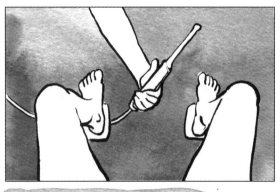

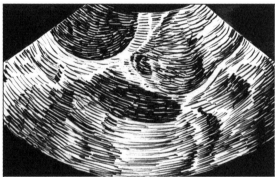

FIVE: DEMONSTRATION BEND

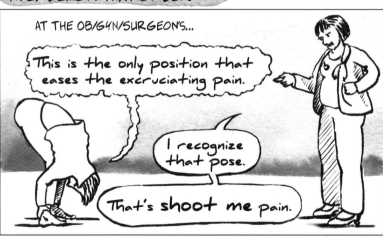

AT THE OB/GYN/SURGEON'S...

This is the only position that eases the excruciating pain.

I recognize that pose.

That's **shoot** me pain.

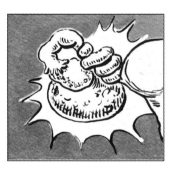

THE CYST HAS CAUSED MY OVARY TO TWIST ON ITS SUPPORTING TISSUES, CUTTING OFF ITS BLOOD SUPPLY.

SIX: MUM

AT THE MEETING TO PLAN THE SURGERY, THE DOCTOR ASKS ME:

> Do you want to keep your uterus if you're having your ovaries removed?

AND I SAY:

> I am not my uterus.

WORDS I WISH SHE HAD QUESTIONED, WORDS I HAVE WANTED TO TAKE BACK EVER SINCE.

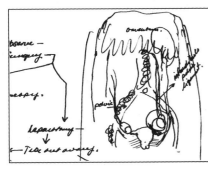

SHE DRAWS A SKETCH OF HOW SHE WILL OPEN ME UP MIDLINE, BECAUSE IT COULD BE CANCER.

SHE WILL TAKE OUT MY OVARIES, TAKE OUT MY UTERUS, AND THEN IF THERE IS VISUAL EVIDENCE OF CANCER SHE WILL DO A COMPLETE PERITONEAL LAVAGE, AND IF NECESSARY REMOVE THE OMENTUM. SHE WILL SEND THE TISSUE SAMPLES TO THE LAB, AND CLOSE ME UP.

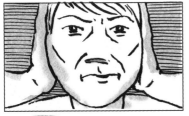
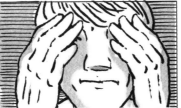
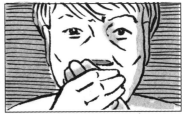

SEVEN: PROSTRATE

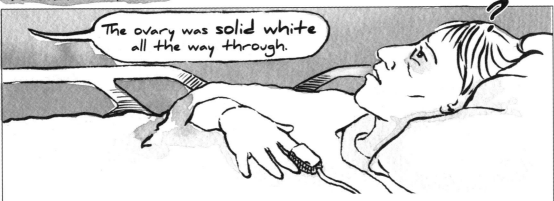

> The ovary was **solid white** all the way through.

THIS STATEMENT PUZZLES ME, BUT SHE SEEMS TO BE TELLING ME THAT THE CYST WAS BENIGN.

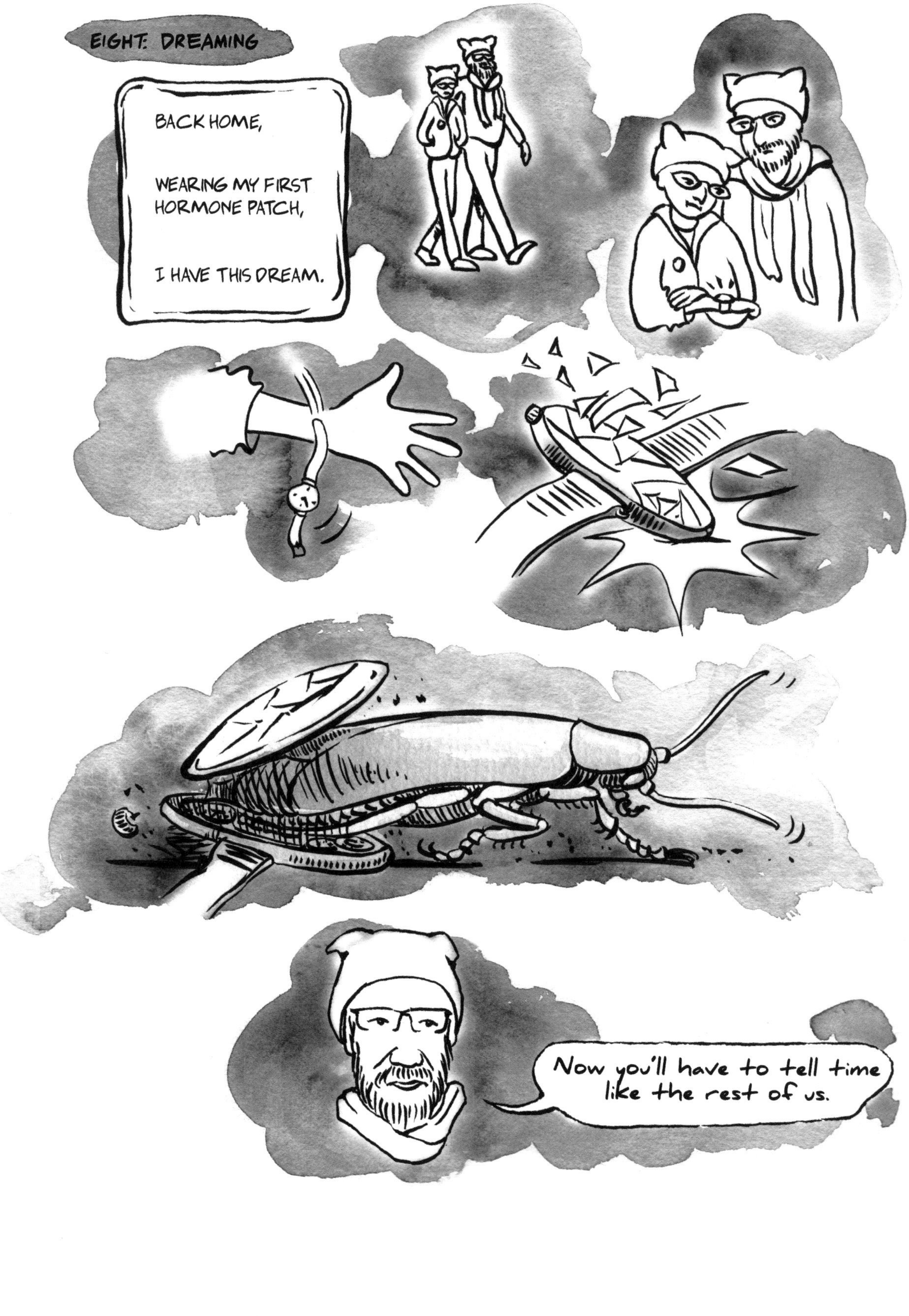
EIGHT: DREAMING
BACK HOME,
WEARING MY FIRST HORMONE PATCH,
I HAVE THIS DREAM.
Now you'll have to tell time like the rest of us.

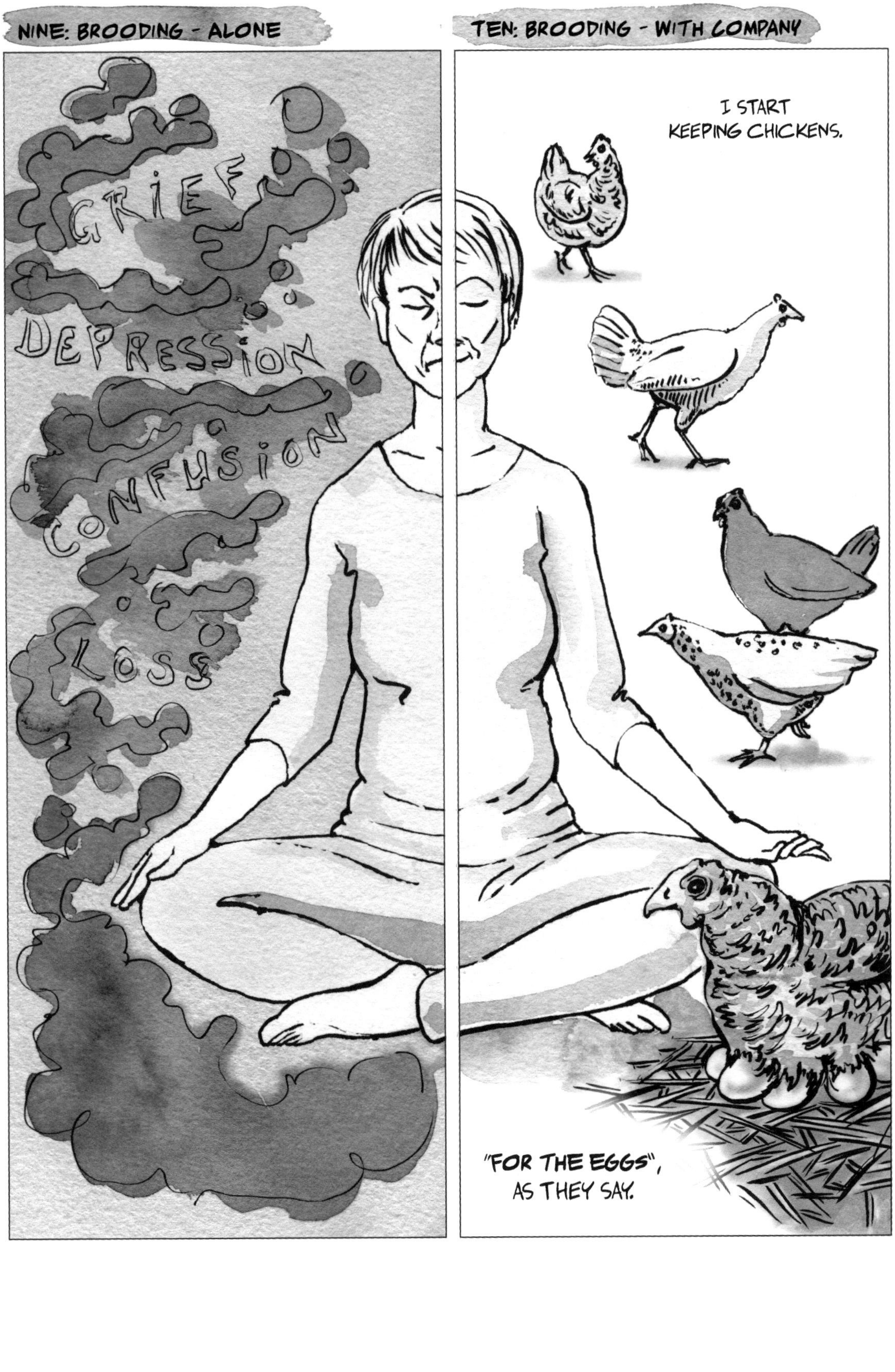
NINE: BROODING - ALONE
GRIEF
DEPRESSION
CONFUSION
LOSS
TEN: BROODING - WITH COMPANY
I START KEEPING CHICKENS.
"FOR THE EGGS", AS THEY SAY.

TODAY ONLY WOMEN'S CARNIVAL
WOW! A CARNIVAL JUST FOR US?
FUNNY... I HAVEN'T HEARD ANYONE TALKING ABOUT THIS...
I DON'T KNOW, MOM...
DON'T BE SO PARANOID, LET'S DO IT!
TICKETS
NO FUN ZONE

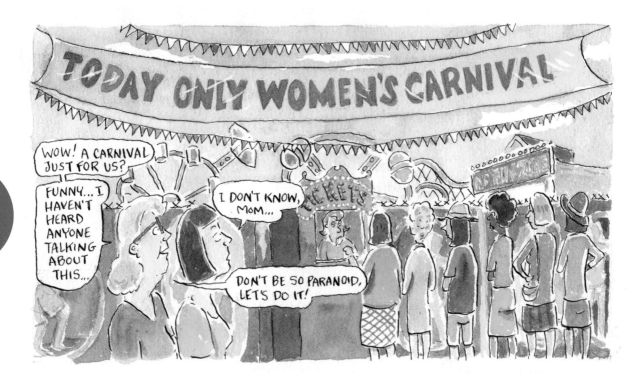

TUNNEL OF LOVE
HERE WE GO!
THIS IS SO CORNY.

THIS IS FUN!
FUNNY... THE WATER'S RED...
ARE WE SINKING?

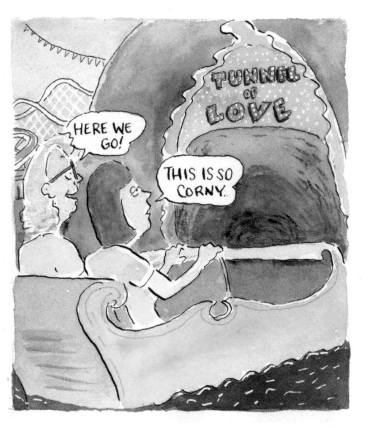

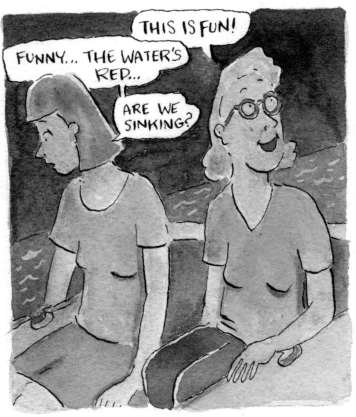

WE'VE STOPPED!
NO MORE RED WATER...
I GUESS WE HAVE TO WALK OUT...
SOME RIDE...

OOH, IT'S SO BRIGHT OUT HERE...
MOM, YOU LOOK DIFFERENT...
I DO? HOW?
...HEY, LOOK!
IT'S A FUNHOUSE!

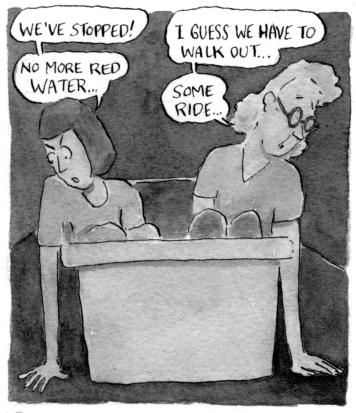

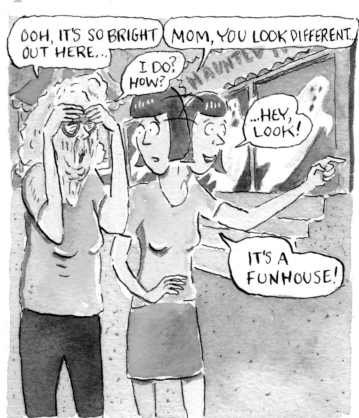

THESE FUNHOUSE MIRRORS ARE HILARIOUS!
HOW COME YOU DON'T LOOK DIFFERENT?

WHOO!
I'M NOT EVEN IN THIS ONE.
I'M INVISIBLE!

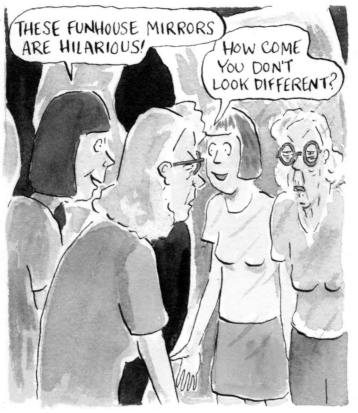

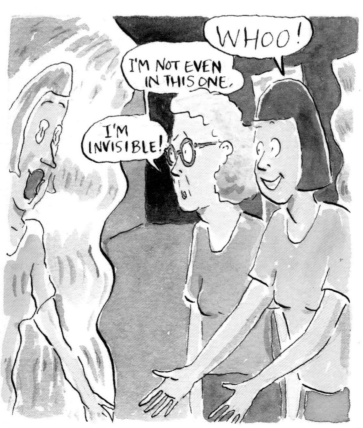

I NEVER LOVED YOUR FATHER!
MOOD
SWING
I LOVE YOUR FATHER SOOOO MUCH!

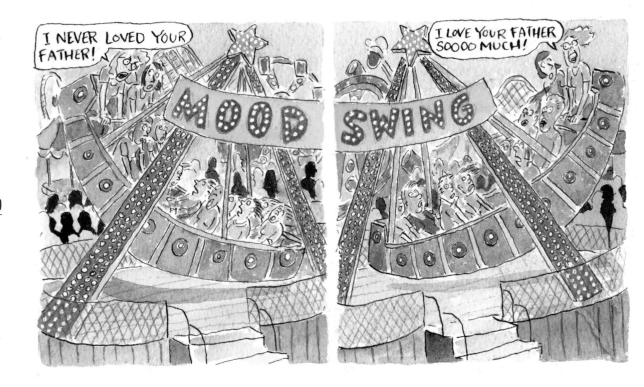

HOT FLASH
FEEL THE
FIERY
OF HELL
THAT ONE WASN'T EVEN FUN...
WHO SAID IT WAS SUPPOSED TO BE?

SHOOTING
OH, LOOK!
I ALWAYS LIKED SHOOTING THOSE DUCKS.
THOSE AREN'T DUCKS, THEY'RE DICKS.
THAT'S RIGHT! EAT LEAD!
WHO'S SORRY NOW, MR. JOHNSON?

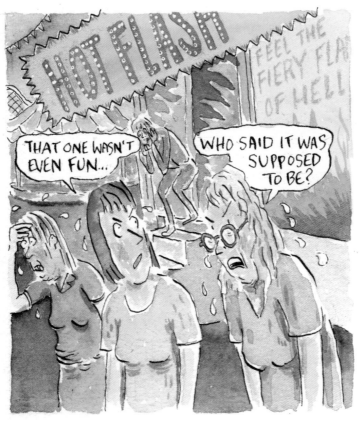

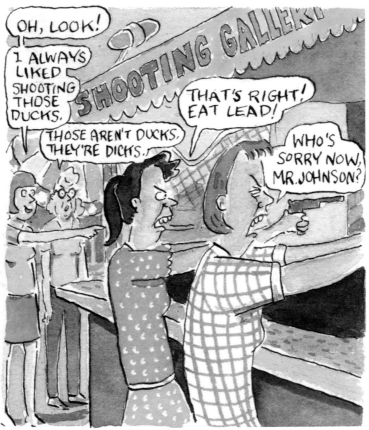

ARCADE
PATRIARCHY
WILL U DIE ALONE?
OOH, PINBALL!

MOM, IS THIS HOW IT WORKS?
R.U. Fertile?
002
153
6612
PRETTY MUCH...
WATCH UR FIGURE DISAPPEAR
BINGO
TWIN BONUS
MATERNAL URGE
CONFLICTING
EMOTIONS
AMBITION DOWN DRAIN

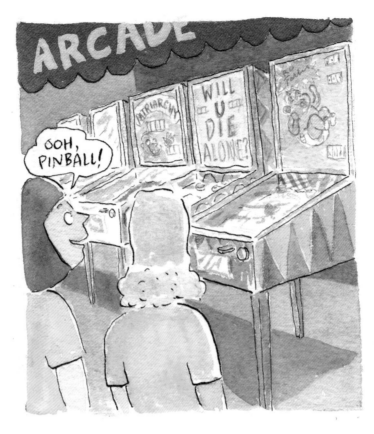

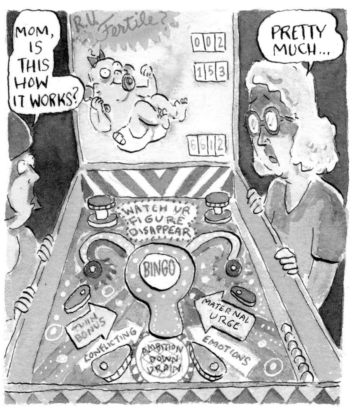

THE HORMONE SCRAMBLER
IS THIS SOME KIND OF METAPHOR?

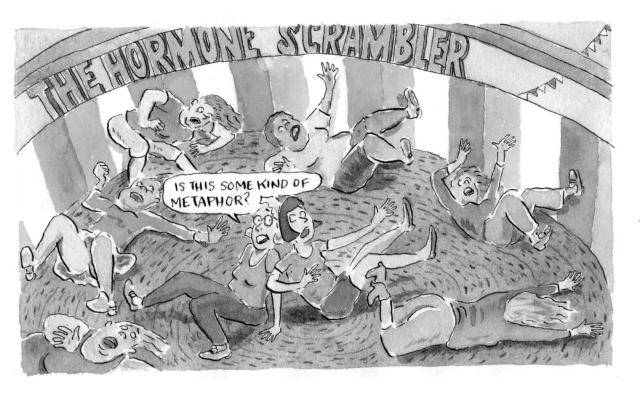

FREAK SHOW
A FREAK SHOW?
IT'S SO POLITICALLY INCORRECT!

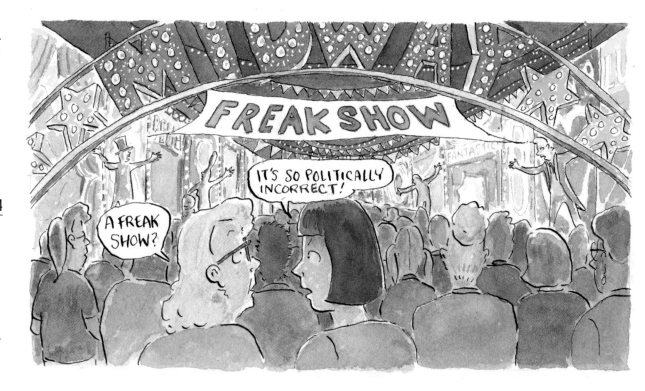

THE WOMAN WHO STILL WEARS THE SAME SIZE PANTS SHE DID IN HIGH SCHOOL
THE WOMAN WHO ASKED FOR A RAISE AND GOT IT!
THE WOM WHO AL GOT EL PRESIDE
SO FAKE!
LADIES, HE ACTUALLY SAID HE WAS SORRY.
HIS NAME WAS GARY.
HEAR THE STORY OF THE WOMAN WHO CONFRONTED HER CO-WORKER!
NO WAY CAN I BUY THAT.

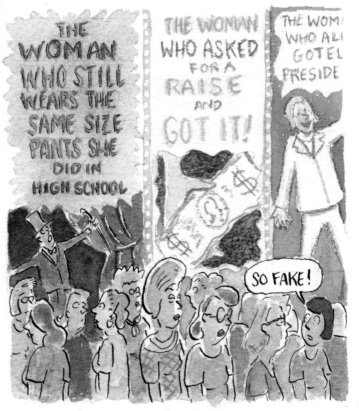

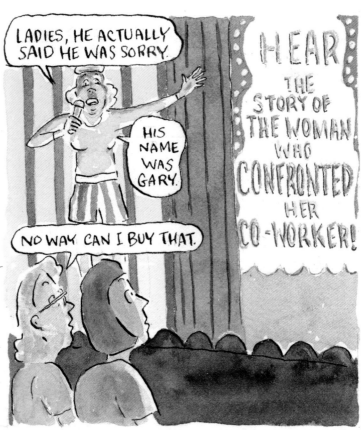

COME SEE THE WORLD'S...
ANGRIEST WOMEN!
SEE THEM GIVE FULL VENT TO YEARS OF PENT-UP RAGE!
SEE HOW THEIR FURY IS HARNESSED TO A GENERATOR POWERING THIS ENTIRE CARNIVAL!
YESSS!
MOM?

YES, FOR ONLY 75 CENTS... THAT'S HOW MUCH A WOMAN MAKES TO EVERY MAN'S DOLLAR...
SEE FOR YOURSELF!
IS IT HORMONES?
OR IS IT RIGHTEOUSLY JUSTIFIED RAGE?
YOU BE THE JUDGE!
TAKE MY MONEY!

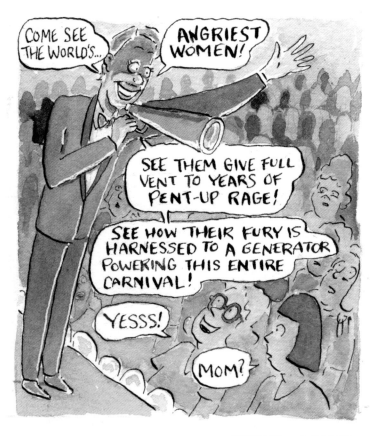

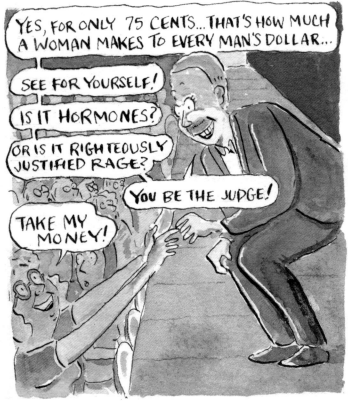

EVERYTHING I'D SAY, THEY'D REPEAT AND TAKE CREDIT!
I REALIZED MY ONLY VALUE WAS AS AN OBJECT!
THEY SAID WOMEN WEREN'T FUNNY!
MY HUSBAND MISPRONOUNCES WORDS JUST TO ANNOY ME!
WHO'S INVISIBLE NOW?

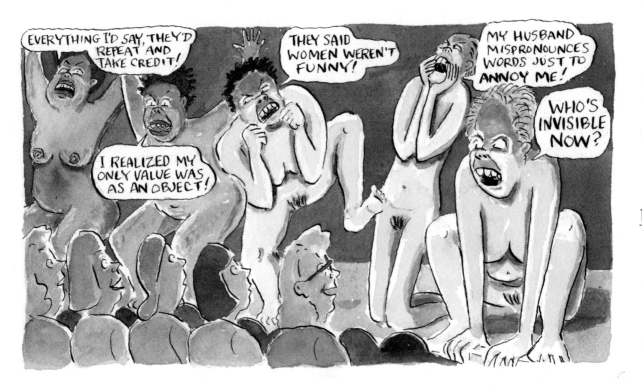

THEY'RE PRETTY CONVINCING...
THEY HAVE SO MUCH POWER!

ONE OF US! ONE OF US! WE ACCEPT YOU, WE ACCEPT YOU, ONE OF US!
THEY'RE TALKING TO YOU, MOM.

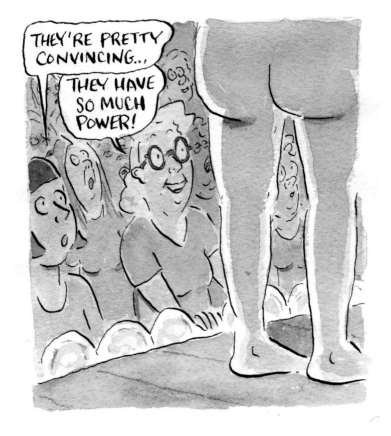

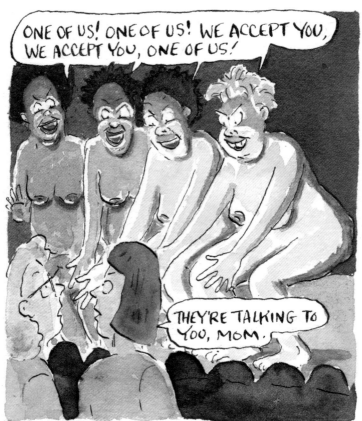

MOM!

I'VE INTERNALIZED MAKING MYSELF SMALLER AND LESSER...
FOR TOO LONG!
WHOOO!
TELL IT!
MOM! IT'S NOT THAT BAD!

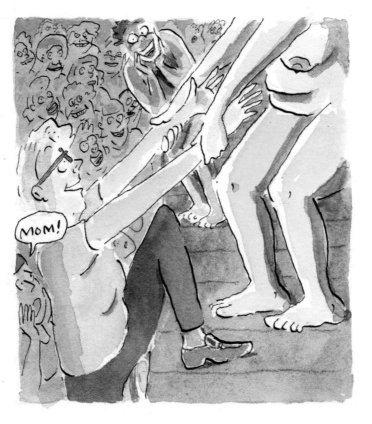

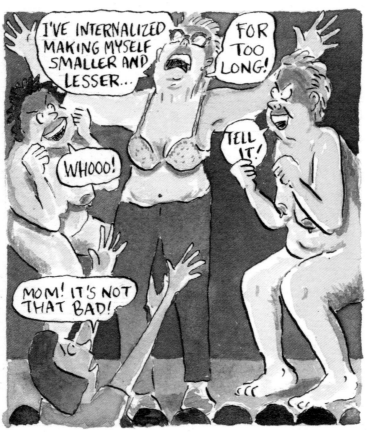

YES IT IS!
I'M NOT COMING HOME!
TELL YOUR FATHER THERE'S A CASSEROLE IN THE-

FUCK THAT!!!

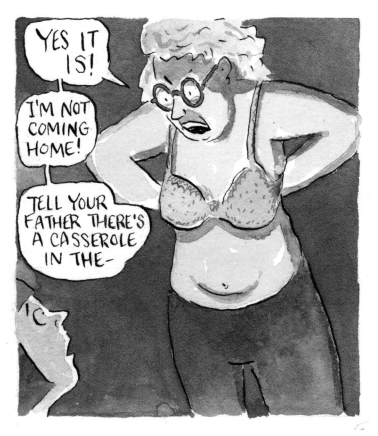

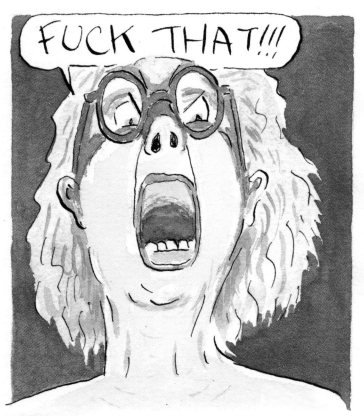

I'M RUNNING AWAY WITH THIS CIRCUS!

ONE DAY YOU WILL TOO!

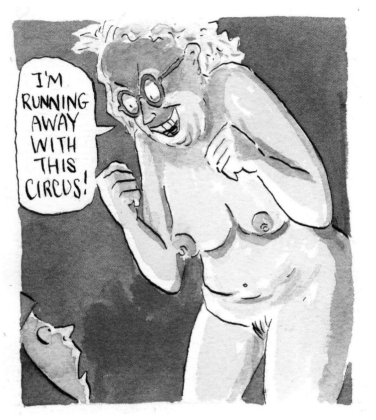

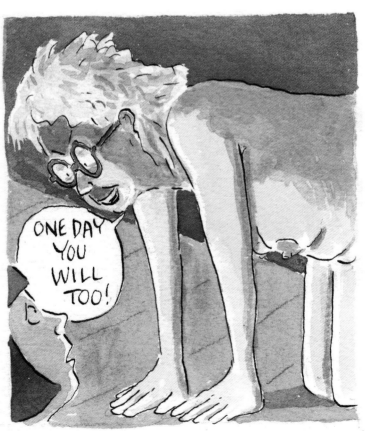

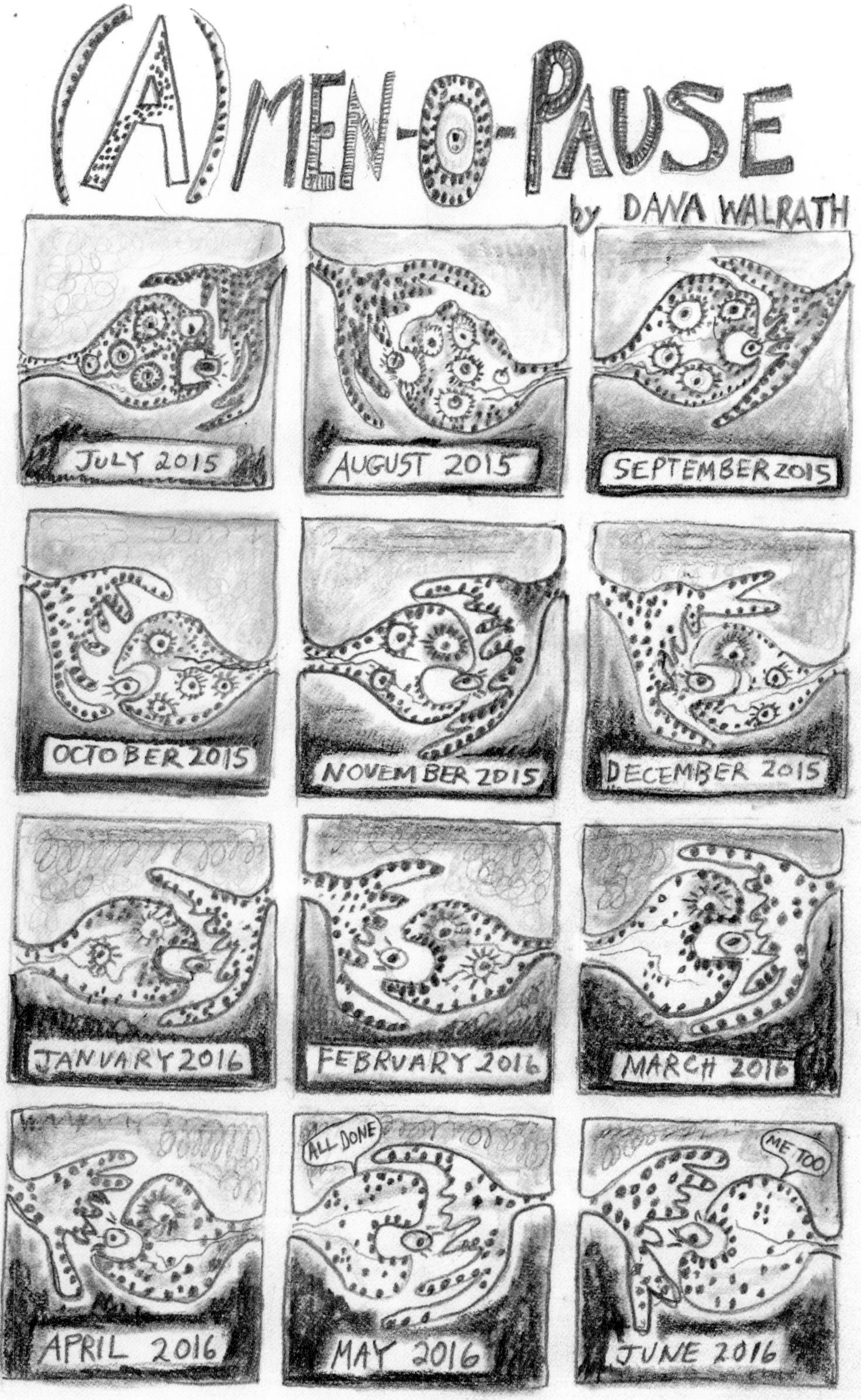
(A)MEN-O-PAUSE
by DANA WALRATH
JULY 2015
AUGUST 2015
SEPTEMBER 2015
OCTOBER 2015
NOVEMBER 2015
DECEMBER 2015
JANUARY 2016
FEBRUARY 2016
MARCH 2016
APRIL 2016
ALL DONE
MAY 2016
ME TOO
JUNE 2016

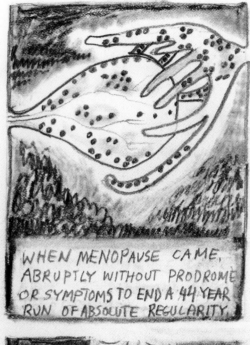

WHEN MENOPAUSE CAME, ABRUPTLY WITHOUT PRODROME OR SYMPTOMS TO END A 44 YEAR RUN OF ABSOLUTE REGULARITY.

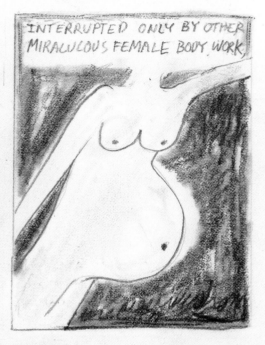

INTERRUPTED ONLY BY OTHER MIRACULOUS FEMALE BODY WORK,

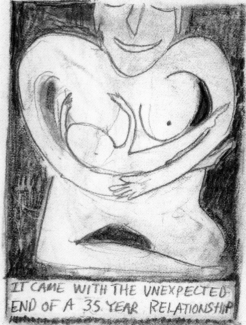

IT CAME WITH THE UNEXPECTED END OF A 35 YEAR RELATIONSHIP

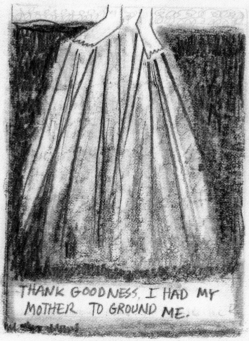

THANK GOODNESS, I HAD MY MOTHER TO GROUND ME.

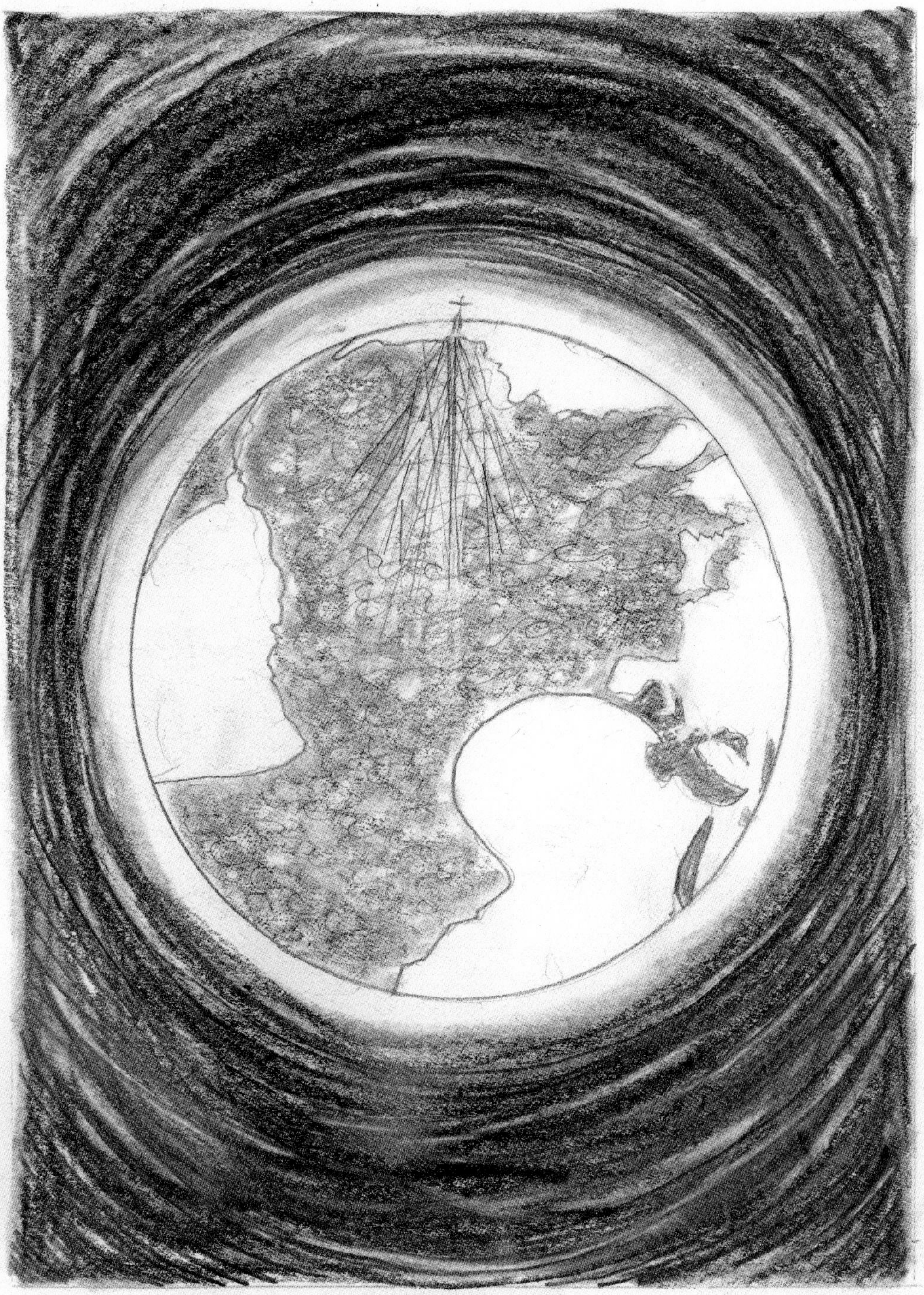

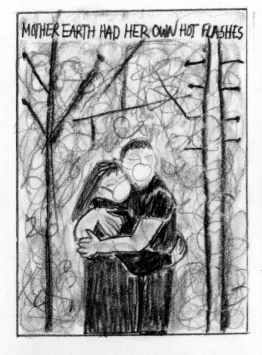

MOTHER EARTH HAD HER OWN HOT FLASHES

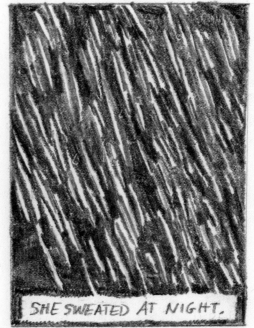

SHE SWEATED AT NIGHT.

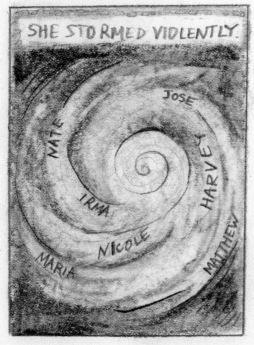

SHE STORMED VIOLENTLY.

JOSE
NATE
HARVEY
IRMA
NICOLE
MARIA
MATTHEW

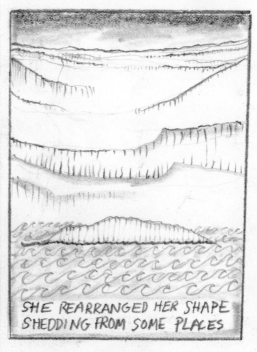

SHE REARRANGED HER SHAPE
SHEDDING FROM SOME PLACES

ADDING TO OTHERS

SHE KNEW HER OWN RADIANCE

AND POWER

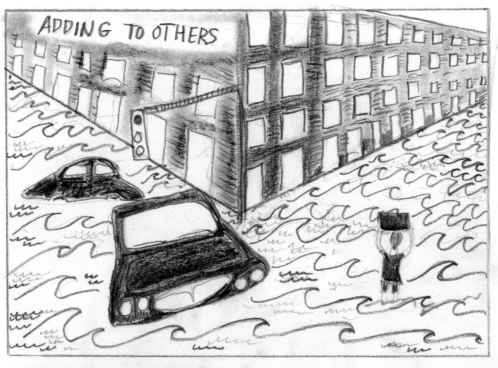

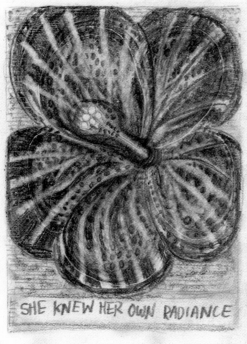

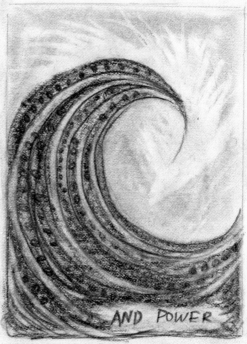

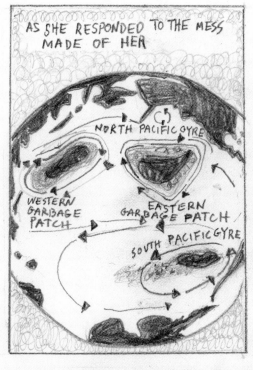

AS SHE RESPONDED TO THE MESS MADE OF HER

NORTH PACIFIC GYRE

WESTERN GARBAGE PATCH

EASTERN GARBAGE PATCH

SOUTH PACIFIC GYRE

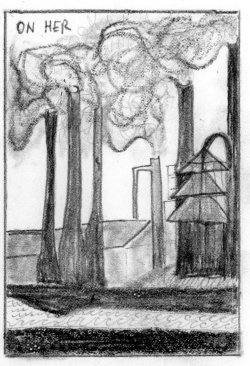

ON HER

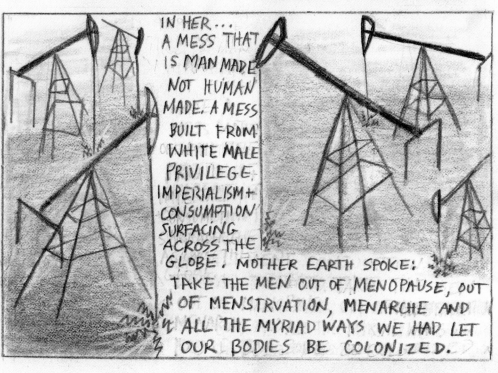

IN HER... A MESS THAT IS MAN MADE NOT HUMAN MADE. A MESS BUILT FROM WHITE MALE PRIVILEGE, IMPERIALISM + CONSUMPTION SURFACING ACROSS THE GLOBE. MOTHER EARTH SPOKE: TAKE THE MEN OUT OF MENOPAUSE, OUT OF MENSTRUATION, MENARCHE AND ALL THE MYRIAD WAYS WE HAD LET OUR BODIES BE COLONIZED.

ON TOP OF THE ENVIRONMENTAL + POLITICAL FOULNESS OF 2016, FOR ME...
GRAB 'EM BY THE PUSSY; YOU CAN DO ANYTHING.
WHATEVER YOU WANT
ACCESS AC
accesshollywood
AMERIC
IT WAS PERSONAL. MY MENOPAUSE COINCIDED WITH HIS CONFESSION
IN 1993...
IN 1999...
IN 1997...
IN 2003... 2007... 2015... ON MONDAY
ALL MY SOULWORK, COMBINED WITH MY TRAINING AS A FEMINIST ANTHROPOLOGIST, PREPARED ME FOR...
THE BLOW, LET ME FATHOM THE SOURCES OF MY OWN BLINDNESS, + CHARTED MY COURSE TO HEALING.

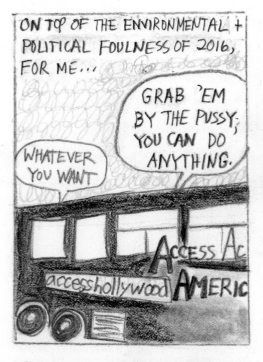

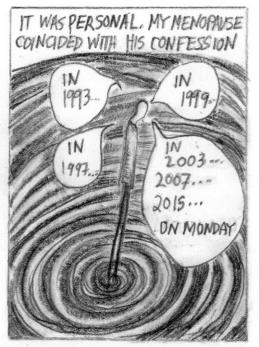

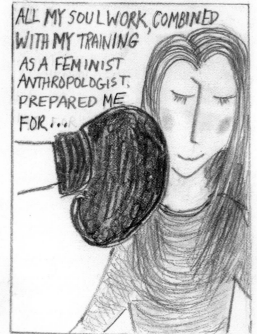

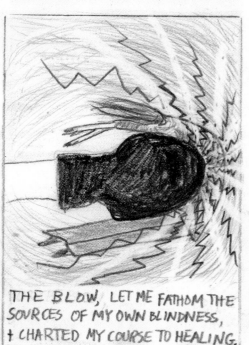

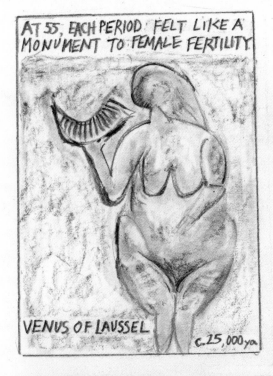

AT 55, EACH PERIOD FELT LIKE A MONUMENT TO FEMALE FERTILITY.

VENUS OF LAUSSEL

c. 25,000 ya

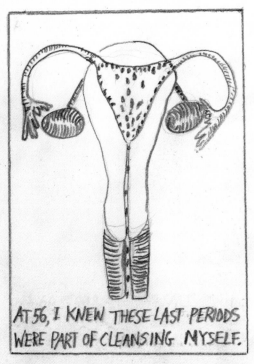

AT 56, I KNEW THESE LAST PERIODS WERE PART OF CLEANSING MYSELF.

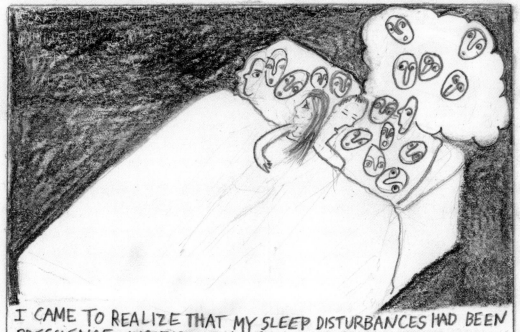

I CAME TO REALIZE THAT MY SLEEP DISTURBANCES HAD BEEN PRESCIENCE INSTEAD OF A PERI-MENOPAUSAL SYMPTOM.

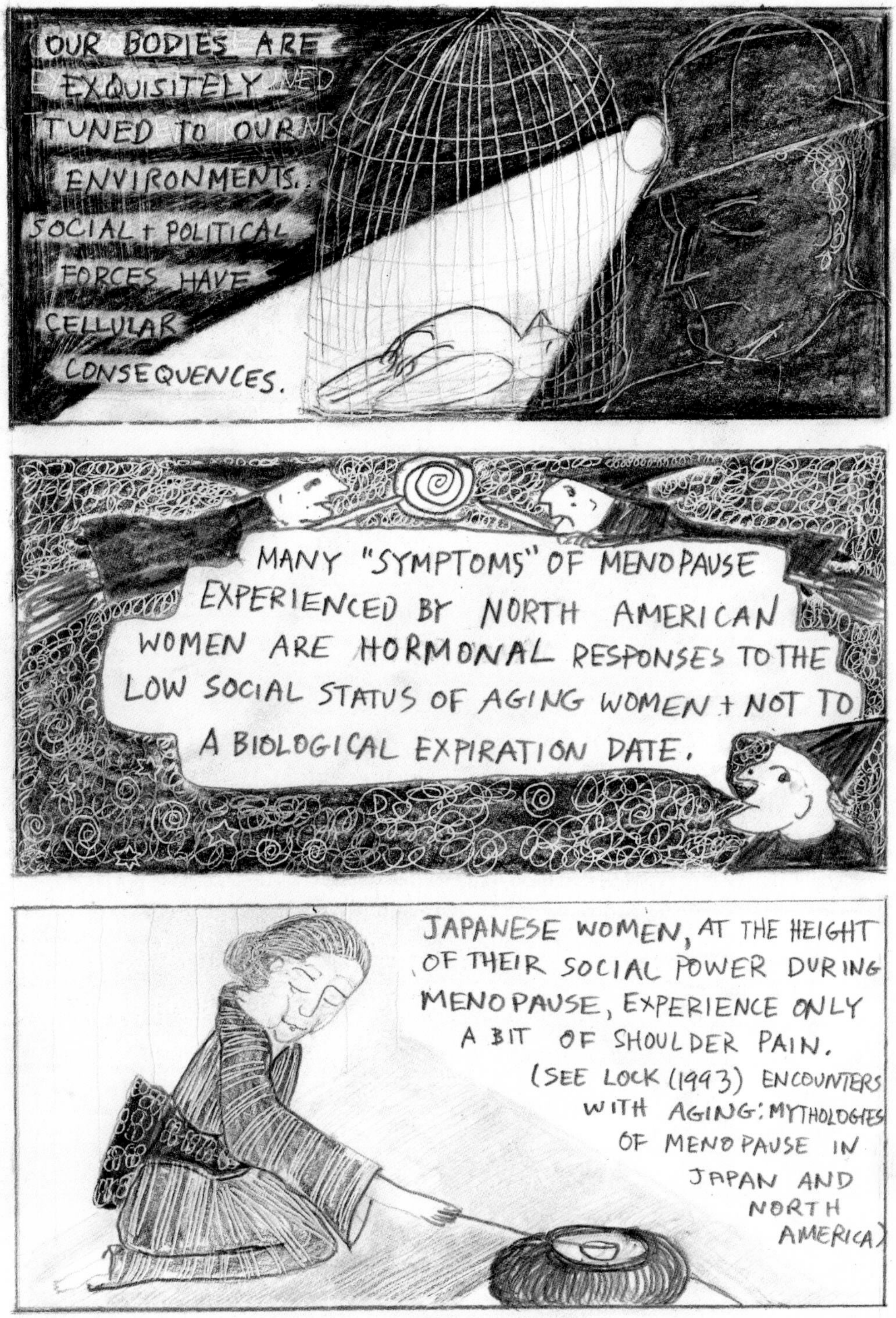
OUR BODIES ARE EXQUISITELY TUNED TO OUR ENVIRONMENTS.
SOCIAL + POLITICAL FORCES HAVE CELLULAR CONSEQUENCES.
MANY "SYMPTOMS" OF MENOPAUSE EXPERIENCED BY NORTH AMERICAN WOMEN ARE HORMONAL RESPONSES TO THE LOW SOCIAL STATUS OF AGING WOMEN + NOT TO A BIOLOGICAL EXPIRATION DATE.
JAPANESE WOMEN, AT THE HEIGHT OF THEIR SOCIAL POWER DURING MENOPAUSE, EXPERIENCE ONLY A BIT OF SHOULDER PAIN.
(SEE LOCK (1993) ENCOUNTERS WITH AGING: MYTHOLOGIES OF MENOPAUSE IN JAPAN AND NORTH AMERICA)

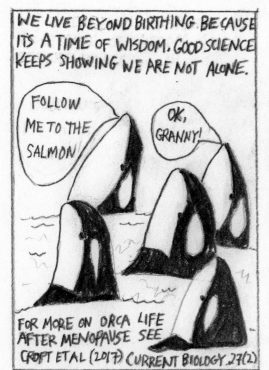

WE LIVE BEYOND BIRTHING BECAUSE IT'S A TIME OF WISDOM. GOOD SCIENCE KEEPS SHOWING WE ARE NOT ALONE.

FOLLOW ME TO THE SALMON

OK, GRANNY!

FOR MORE ON ORCA LIFE AFTER MENOPAUSE SEE CROFT ET AL (2017) CURRENT BIOLOGY 27(2)

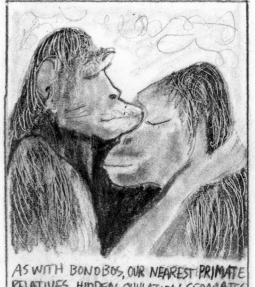

AS WITH BONOBOS, OUR NEAREST PRIMATE RELATIVES, HIDDEN OVULATION SEPARATES SEXUALITY FROM REPRODUCTION. PHYSICAL CONNECTION CREATES BONDS BEYOND OWNERSHIP + GENETIC RELATEDNESS + PATRIARCHAL NOTIONS OF SPREADING SEED.

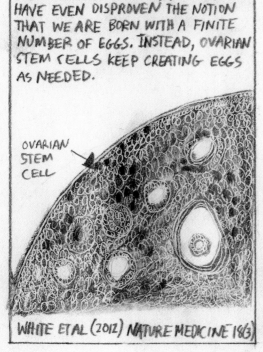

OVER THE PAST DECADE, BIOLOGISTS HAVE EVEN DISPROVEN THE NOTION THAT WE ARE BORN WITH A FINITE NUMBER OF EGGS. INSTEAD, OVARIAN STEM CELLS KEEP CREATING EGGS AS NEEDED.

OVARIAN STEM CELL

WHITE ET AL (2012) NATURE MEDICINE 18(3)

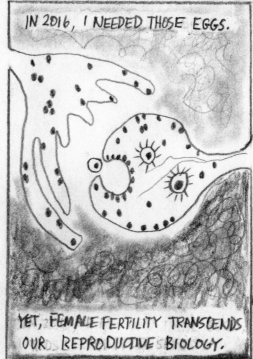

IN 2016, I NEEDED THOSE EGGS.

YET, FEMALE FERTILITY TRANSCENDS OUR REPRODUCTIVE BIOLOGY.

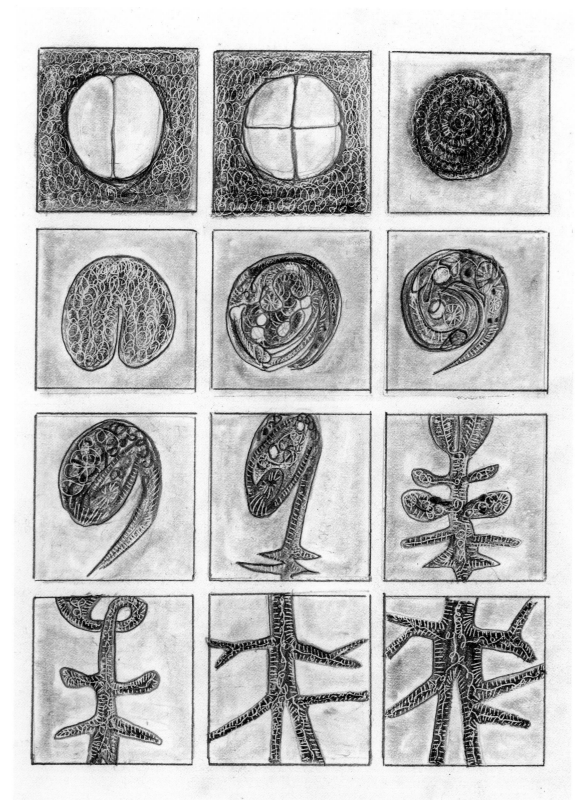

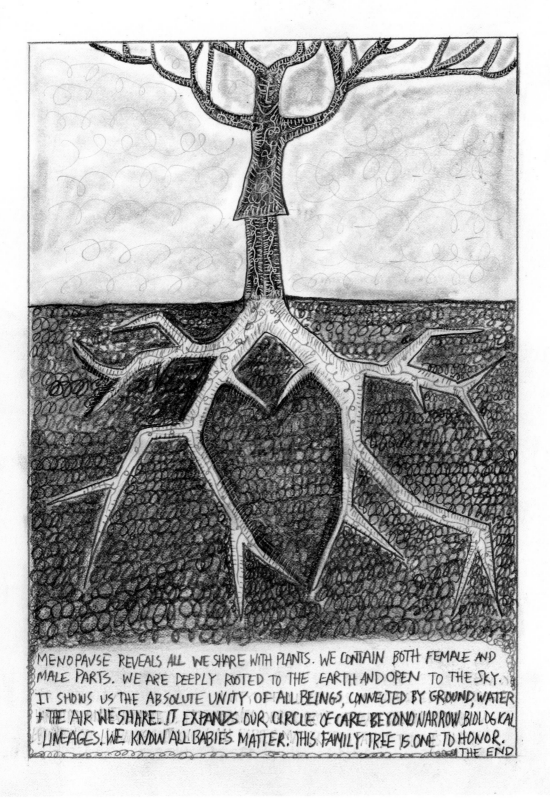

MENOPAUSE REVEALS ALL WE SHARE WITH PLANTS. WE CONTAIN BOTH FEMALE AND MALE PARTS. WE ARE DEEPLY ROOTED TO THE EARTH AND OPEN TO THE SKY. IT SHOWS US THE ABSOLUTE UNITY OF ALL BEINGS, CONNECTED BY GROUND, WATER + THE AIR WE SHARE. IT EXPANDS OUR CIRCLE OF CARE BEYOND NARROW BIOLOGICAL LINEAGES! WE KNOW ALL BABIES MATTER. THIS FAMILY TREE IS ONE TO HONOR.
THE END

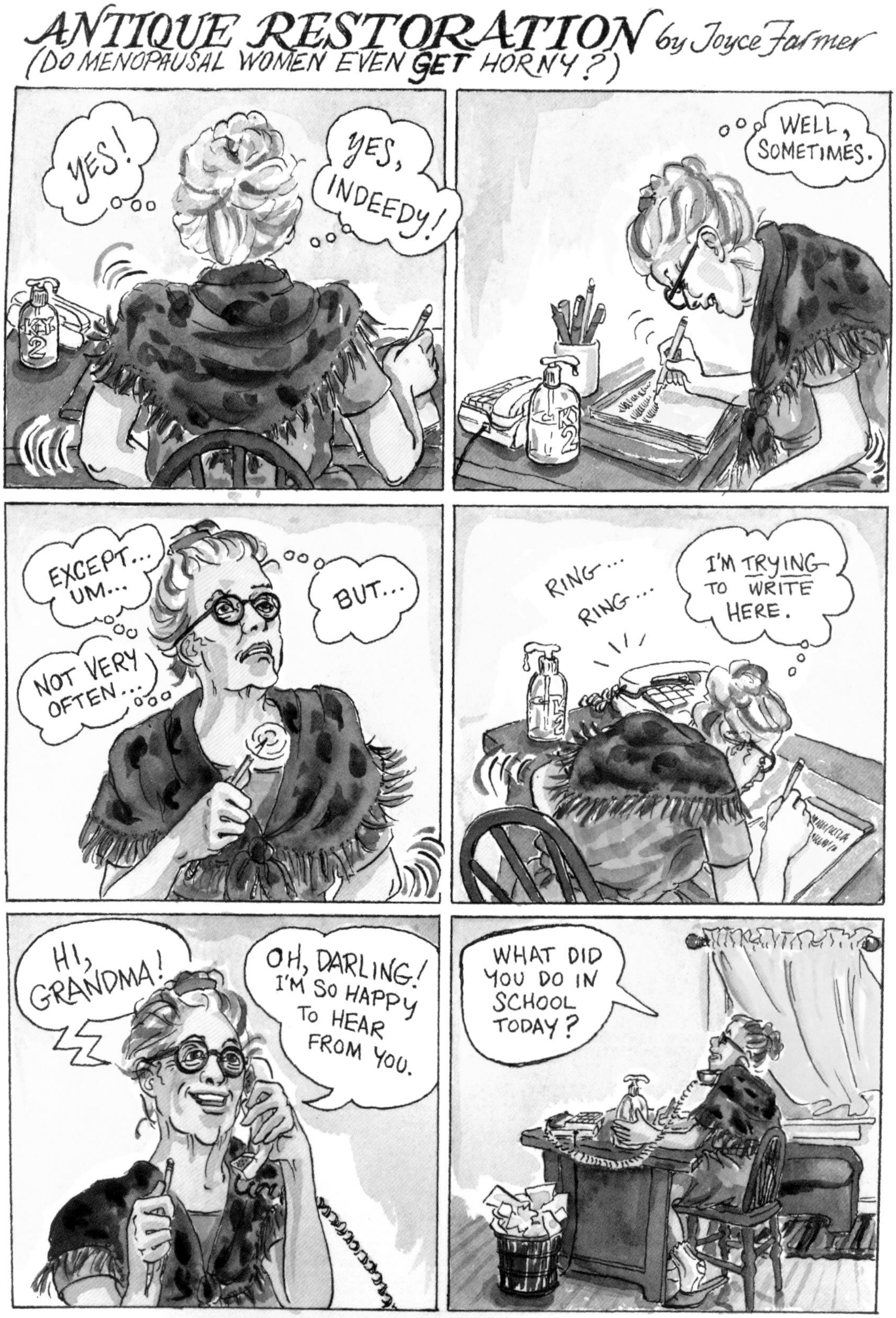
ANTIQUE RESTORATION by Joyce Farmer
(DO MENOPAUSAL WOMEN EVEN GET HORNY?)
YES!
YES, INDEEDY!
WELL, SOMETIMES.
EXCEPT... UM...
NOT VERY OFTEN...
BUT...
RING... RING...
I'M TRYING TO WRITE HERE.
HI, GRANDMA!
OH, DARLING! I'M SO HAPPY TO HEAR FROM YOU.
WHAT DID YOU DO IN SCHOOL TODAY?

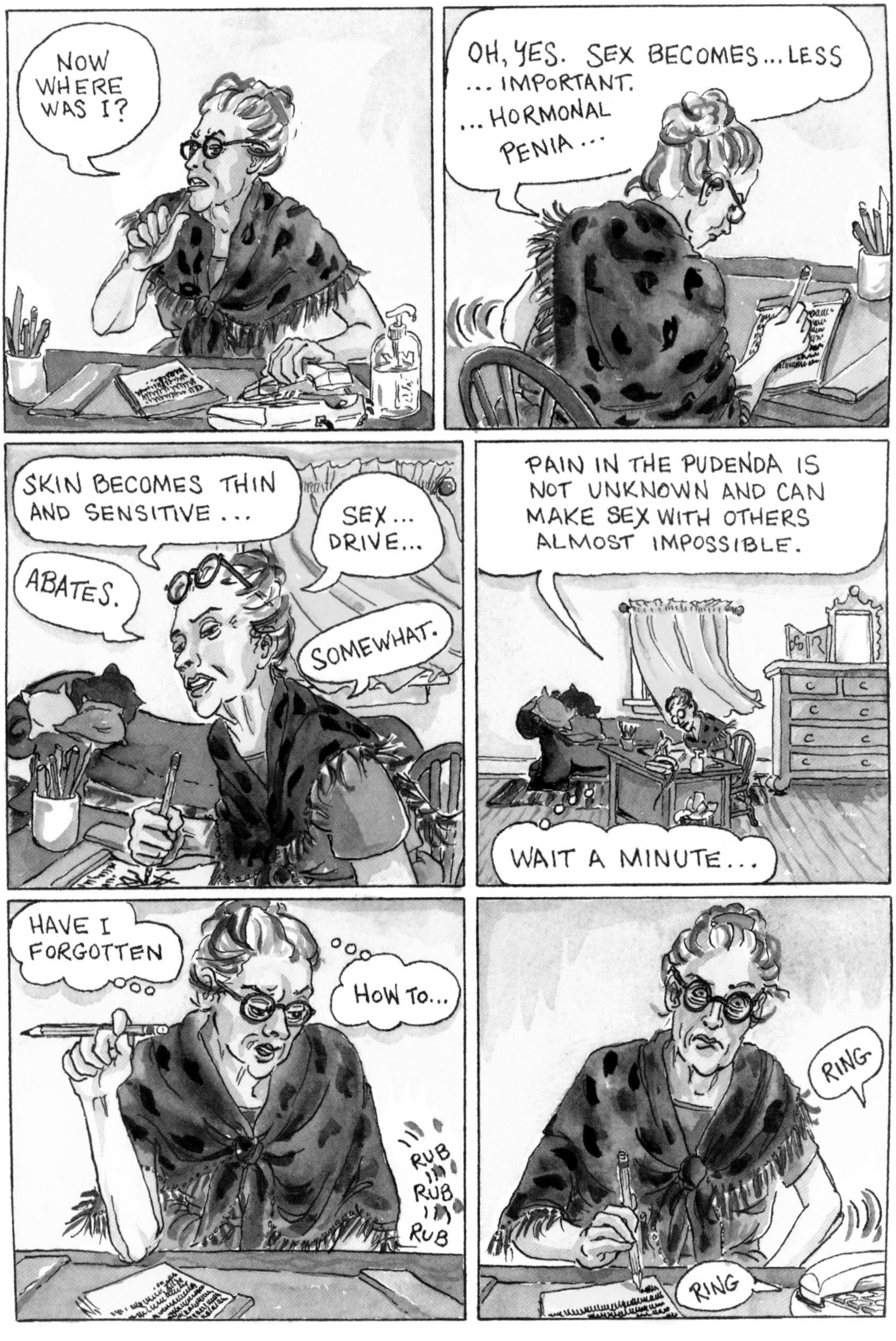
NOW WHERE WAS I?
OH, YES. SEX BECOMES... LESS ... IMPORTANT. ... HORMONAL PENIA ...
SKIN BECOMES THIN AND SENSITIVE ...
SEX... DRIVE...
ABATES.
SOMEWHAT.
PAIN IN THE PUDENDA IS NOT UNKNOWN AND CAN MAKE SEX WITH OTHERS ALMOST IMPOSSIBLE.
WAIT A MINUTE...
HAVE I FORGOTTEN
HOW TO...
RUB RUB RUB
RING
RING

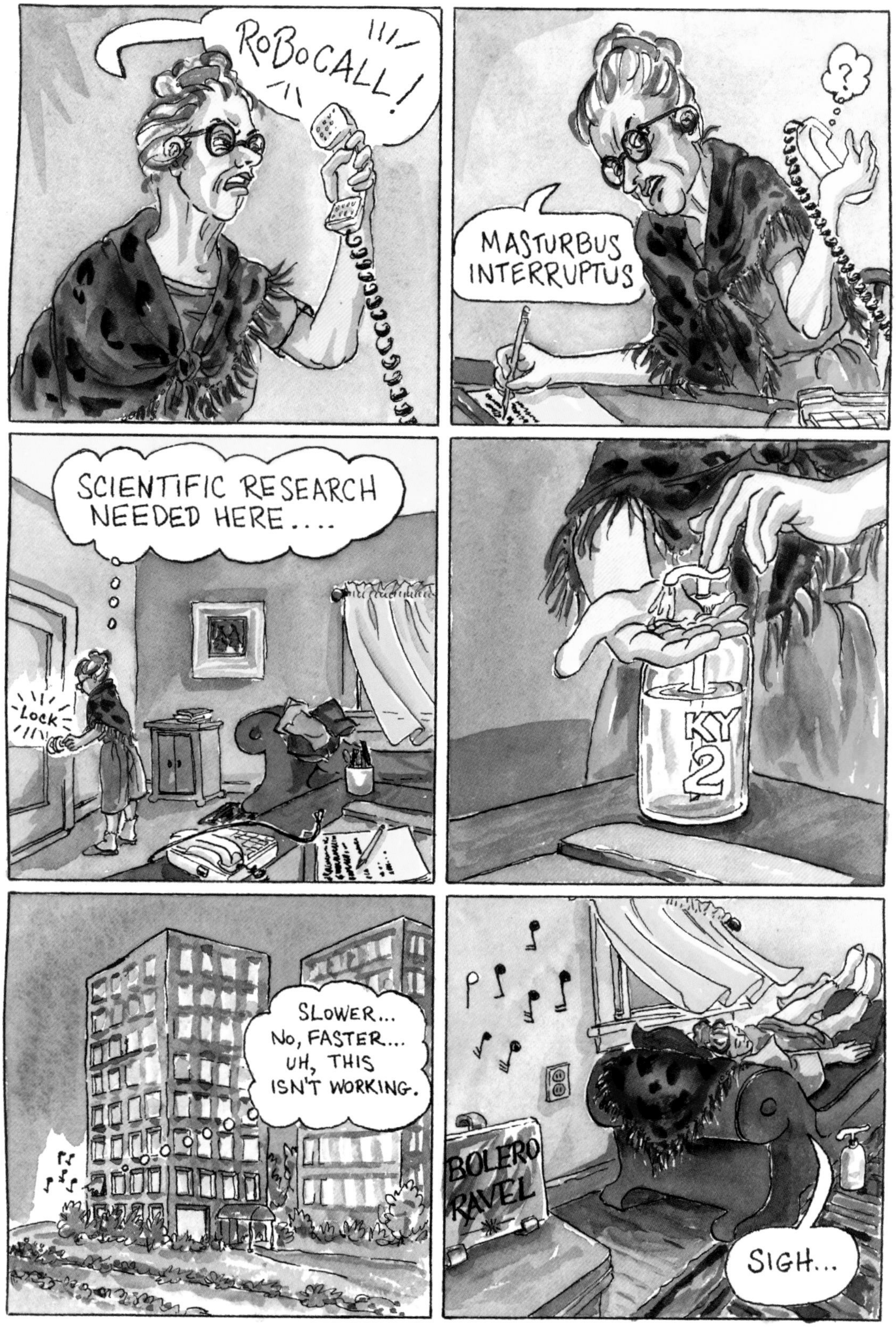
ROBOCALL!
MASTURBUS INTERRUPTUS
?
SCIENTIFIC RESEARCH NEEDED HERE....
LOCK
KY 2
SLOWER... No, FASTER... UH, THIS ISN'T WORKING.
BOLERO RAVEL
SIGH...

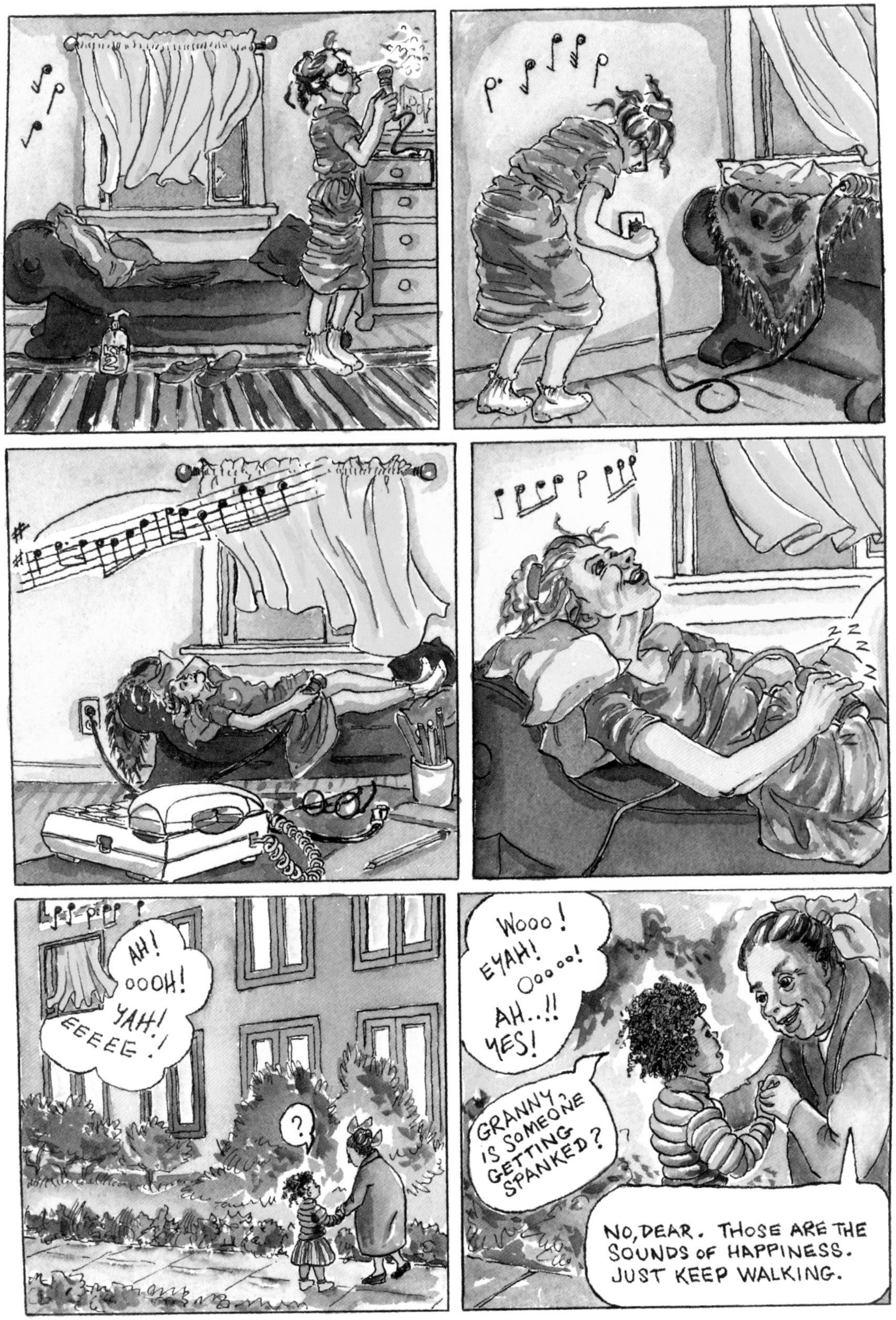
AH! OOOH! YAH! EEEEE!
?
WOOO! EYAH! OOOOO! AH..!! YES!
GRANNY, IS SOMEONE GETTING SPANKED?
NO, DEAR. THOSE ARE THE SOUNDS OF HAPPINESS. JUST KEEP WALKING.

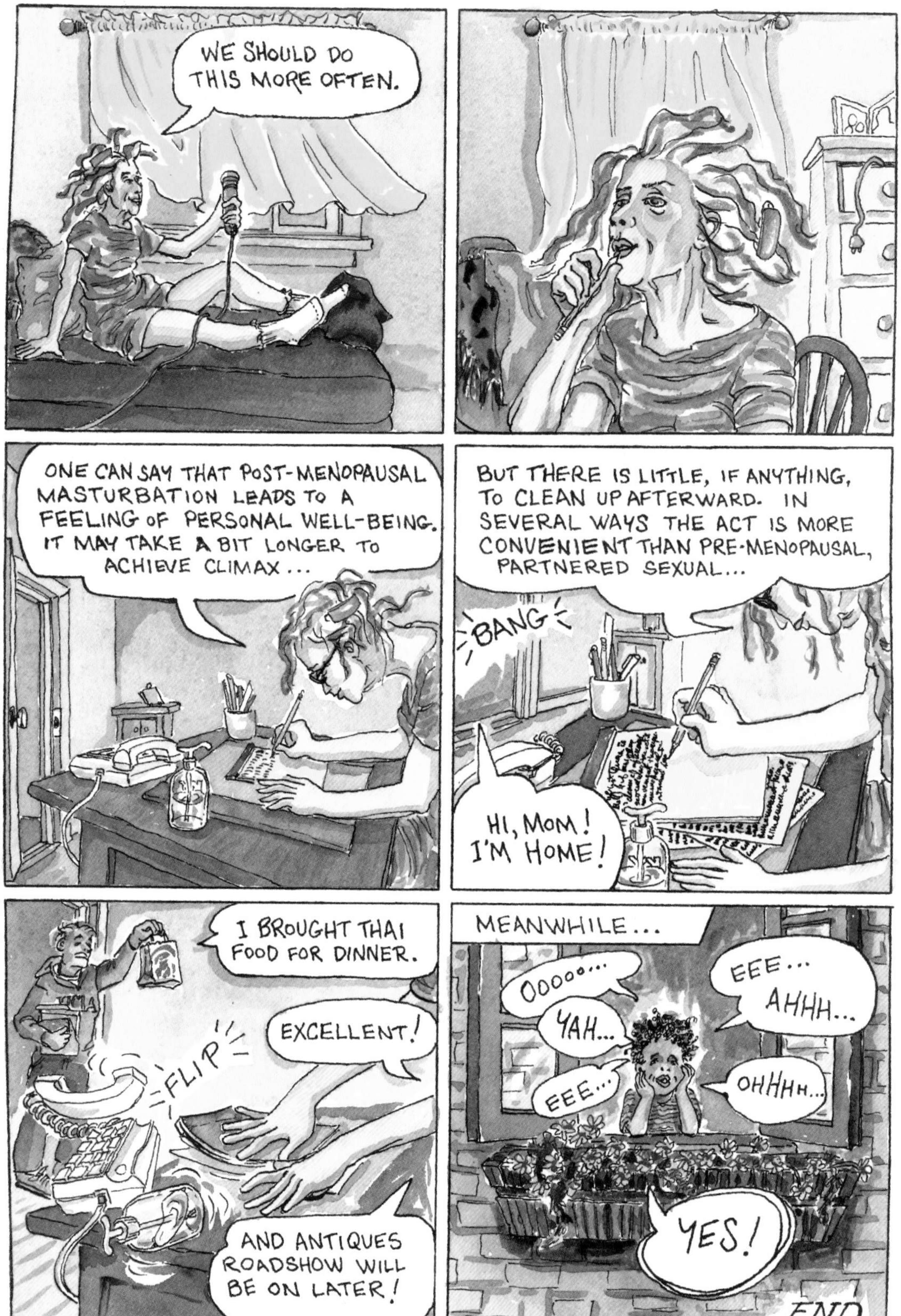
WE SHOULD DO THIS MORE OFTEN.
ONE CAN SAY THAT POST-MENOPAUSAL MASTURBATION LEADS TO A FEELING OF PERSONAL WELL-BEING. IT MAY TAKE A BIT LONGER TO ACHIEVE CLIMAX ...
BUT THERE IS LITTLE, IF ANYTHING, TO CLEAN UP AFTERWARD. IN SEVERAL WAYS THE ACT IS MORE CONVENIENT THAN PRE-MENOPAUSAL, PARTNERED SEXUAL...
BANG
HI, MOM! I'M HOME!
I BROUGHT THAI FOOD FOR DINNER.
FLIP
EXCELLENT!
AND ANTIQUES ROADSHOW WILL BE ON LATER!
MEANWHILE...
OOOOO...
YAH...
EEE...
EEE... AHHH...
OHHHH...
YES!
END

resources

Books

Davies, Sasha, Nancy Nowacek, and Kate Bingaman-Burt. *Menopause: An Imperfect Guide*. 2017. https://www.sashadavies.com/menopauseanimperfectprimer.

Foxcroft, Louise. *Hot Flushes, Cold Science: A History of the Modern Menopause*. London: Granta, 2009.

Goldsworthy, Joanna, ed. *Certain Age: Reflecting on the Menopause*. London: Virago Press, 1993.

Houck, Judith A. *Hot and Bothered: Women, Medicine, and Menopause in Modern America*. Cambridge: Harvard University Press, 2006.

Articles

Davis, Lisa Selin. "Puberty for the Middle Age." *New York Times*, November 19, 2018. https://www.nytimes.com/2018/11/19/opinion/symptomsperimenopausemenopausemiddleage.html.

George, Rose. "It Feels Like Derangement: Menopause, Depression, & Me." *New York Review of Books*, August 8, 2018. https://www.nybooks.com/daily/2018/08/08/itfeelslikeaderangementmenopausedepressionme.

Renkl, Margaret. "The Gift of Menopause." *New York Times*, August 5, 2018. https://www.nytimes.com/2018/08/05/opinion/thegiftofmenopause.html.

Online

"How to Survive Menopause." *Unladylike* (podcast), episode 18, June 26, 2018. https://unladylike.co/episodes/018/menopause.

Michel, Karen. "My Dinner with Menopause." PRX, January 1, 1996. https://beta.prx.org/stories/6790.

The North American Menopause Society, http://www.menopause.org

Renee, Lisa. "The Long Middle." *Medium*. https://medium.com/s/thelongmiddle.

"Unraveling." *The Bodies* (podcast), episode 8, October 17, 2018. https://www.bodiespodcast.com/resourcepages/2018/8/28/episode3anxiousmessmxm4rsb32fn5w6s.

contributors

Lynda Barry is the creator of *Ernie Pook's Comeek*, which was syndicated in alternative weeklies for three decades. She is the author of *The Freddie Stories*; *One! Hundred! Demons!*; *The! Greatest! of! Marlys!*; *Cruddy: An Illustrated Novel*; *Naked Ladies! Naked Ladies! Naked Ladies!*; and *The Good Times Are Killing Me*, which was adapted as an off-Broadway play. She has written four best-selling and acclaimed creative how-to graphic novels: *What It Is* (which won the Eisner Award for Best Reality Based Graphic Novel); *Picture This*; *Syllabus: Notes From an Accidental Professor*; and *Making Comics*. She lives in Wisconsin, where she is the Chazen Family Distinguished Chair in Art at the University of Wisconsin–Madison. Lynda is also a 2019 recipient of a MacArthur Fellowship.

Maureen Burdock was born in the Black Forest in Germany in 1970. She grew up during the Cold War Era in Germany and the United States. Her creative and scholarly work examines topics of displacement, gender, memory, and trauma. Burdock is currently working on *The Baroness of Have-Nothing*, a graphic memoir that is her dissertation in the Cultural Studies PhD Program at the University of California, Davis. Before working toward her PhD, she earned an MFA in Studio Art and an MA in Visual and Critical Studies from the California College of the Arts in San Francisco. Burdock is the creator of *Feminist Fables for the Twenty-first Century: The F Word Project* (2015), a series of graphic fables that address forms of gender-based violence in several cultures.

Jennifer Camper's collections of comics include *Rude Girls and Dangerous Women* and *subGURLZ*. She edited two *Juicy Mother* comics anthologies. Her work appears in numerous publications, comic books, and anthologies and has been exhibited internationally. She is the founding director of the biennial Queers & Comics Conference. jennifercamper.com.

KC Councilor is a transgender cartoonist and an assistant professor of communication at Southern Connecticut State University. You can see more of his work at kccouncilor.com.

Leslie Ewing has worked to further LGBTQ civil rights for over thirty years. She recently retired after leading the Pacific Center for Human Growth in Berkeley, California, as its executive director for over ten years. Leslie has been a cartoonist for most of her life. Her strip *Mid-Dyke Crisis* ran in LGBTQ periodicals between 1985 and 2001. Her cartoons have also appeared in *Wimmin's Comix* and *Gay Comix*. Her cartoons chronicle the evolution of the women's liberation movement and the role of women during the AIDS and breast cancer pandemics. www.leslieewing.com.

Joyce Farmer is an American cartoonist and major participant in the underground comics movement. With Lyn Chevli she created and published the first all-women's comic book, *Tits and Clits Comix*, in 1972. In 2011, her graphic novel *Special Exits* won the National Cartoonists Society's Reuben Award and was nominated for an Eisner Award.

Ellen Forney is the author of the best-selling graphic memoirs *Marbles: Mania, Depression, Michelangelo, and Me* and *Rock Steady: Brilliant Advice from My Bipolar Life*. She curated *Graphic Medicine: Ill-Conceived & Well-Drawn*, a traveling exhibition for the National Library of Medicine, and teaches comics at Cornish College of the Arts in Seattle. www.ellenforney.com.

Ann M. Fox is a professor of English at Davidson College specializing in modern and contemporary drama, disability studies in literature and art, and graphic medicine. Her scholarship on disability, drama, and art has been published widely, and she has co-curated four disability-related visual arts exhibitions.

Keet Geniza is a Filipina cartoonist, illustrator, and zinester living in Toronto, Canada, where she is always keeping an eye out for stylish grandmas to draw in her sketchbook.

Roberta Gregory's unique comics have been in print since the 1970s. She has a wide variety of work but is best known for her Bitchy Bitch character, star of forty issues of Roberta's *Naughty Bits* series as well as stage and animated incarnations. Her latest book is *True Cat Toons*. The comic included here was originally published in *Naughty Bits* #40. www.robertagregory.com.

Teva Harrison is the author of the best-selling, award-winning, critically acclaimed hybrid graphic memoir *In-Between Days: A Memoir About Living with Cancer*, where this piece originally appeared. She also created *The Joyful Living Colouring Book* and *Not One of These Poems Is About You*. Teva regularly spoke on creativity and led workshops on telling life stories. Teva died in April 2019 of breast cancer. www.tevaharrison.com.

Rachael House is an artist who makes events, objects, performances, drawings, and zines. She exhibits inside and away from gallery spaces, locally and internationally. In the 1990s her autobiographical comic zine *Red Hanky Panky* was part of a thriving UK queerzine scene. She enjoys smashing the patriarchy and making zines about her punk rock menopause. Rachael lives with her lover and a very splendid cat. www.rachaelhouse.com; @rachaellhouse.

Leah Jones lives in Chicago, where she dabbles in stand-up comedy, calls her senators to protect the Affordable Care Act, and is active in the Jewish community. She has an MS in health communications from Northwestern University and recently opened her own consultancy called Natiiv Facilitation.

Monica Lalanda is a Spanish emergency-medicine doctor and medical cartoonist. She has a special interest in health communication and has completed two MSc degrees in medical ethics. Monica has published *Con-ciencia Médica*, the Spanish Medical Ethics Code in comic form. She also is a founder and co-manager of medicinagrafica.com, a Spanish-language sister site to GraphicMedicine.org, and hosted the 2018 and 2019 Congreso de Medicina Gráfica in Zaragoza, Spain. monicalalanda.com.

Cathy Leamy is a cartoonist and health communication specialist from Boston. She's also a member of the comics collective Boston Comics Roundtable. When she's not cartooning, Cathy is probably gawking at gross clinical stuff or watching wrestling. www.metrokitty.com.

Ajuan Mance is a visual artist and a professor of English at Mills College in Oakland, California. In her comics and zines, she uses humor to explore the complexities of race, gender, and power in the contemporary United States. She is the creator of *Gender Studies*, an autobiographical comic series that recounts her humorous adventures as a Black nerd navigating the complexities of gender.

Jessica Moran has always had a passion for the arts. That, and her interest in movies and filmmaking, spurred her to complete the Algonquin College Animation program in 2017. Since then, she has worked as a layout artist for Mercury Filmworks, most notably on the *Tangled* series. Her personal artwork covers a wide range of projects, including character art, portraits, and various pop-culture pieces. She lives in Ottawa, Ontario.

Mimi Pond is the author of the recent graphic novels *Over Easy* and *The Customer Is Always Wrong*, about her sordid waitressing career in late 1970s Oakland, California. She lives in Los Angeles and is developing an animated TV series about a beauty school and a graphic novel about Britain's famous Mitford Sisters. Her comic was commissioned for and originally appeared at www.topic.com. www.mimipond.com.

Sharon Rosenzweig became a cartoonist after a decade of teaching painting and printmaking at the School of the Art Institute of Chicago. She and her husband, Aaron Freeman, co-created *The Comic Torah*. Her cartoons and comics have appeared in *Harper's Magazine*, the *Huffington Post*, *Cartoon Movement*, and the *Annals of Internal Medicine*. Her comic "Judgment Call" was selected as a Notable Comic for *The Best American Comics 2018*. sharonrosenzweig.blogspot.com.

Joyce Schachter is the program director of the Urogynecology and Reconstructive Pelvic Surgery Fellowship in the Department of Obstetrics and Gynecology at The Ottawa Hospital, Ottawa, Ontario, Canada.

Susan M. Squier is Brill Professor Emerita of English and Women's, Gender, and Sexuality Studies at Penn State University and an Einstein Visiting Fellow at the Freie Universität, Berlin, where she is part of the PathoGraphics project. When she experienced the surgical menopause that appears in the comic she co-created with Shelley Wall, she was researching and writing *Liminal Lives: Imagining the Human at the Frontiers of Biomedicine*. Her other books include *Poultry Science, Chicken Culture: A Partial Alphabet* and *Graphic Medicine Manifesto* (co-authored with Czerwiec, Williams, Green, Myers, and Smith). Her co-edited volume with Irmela Marei Krüger-Fürhoff, *PathoGraphics: Narrative, Aesthetics, Contention, Community*, is forthcoming from Penn State Press in 2020 in the Graphic Medicine series. www.susanmerrillsquier.com.

Emily Steinberg is a painter and graphic novelist. She has shown her work in the United States and Europe. Most recently, she has been named Humanities Scholar in Residence at Drexel College of Medicine, where she will teach medical students how to draw their own stories in words and images. She earned her MFA and BFA from the University of Pennsylvania and is currently a lecturer in fine art at Penn State Abington. emilysteinberg.com.

Dr. Nicola Streeten is a speaker, writer, drawer, teacher of comics, and organizer of comics events. She has worked nationally and internationally in a wide range of contexts and with a diverse variety of people. Her graphic memoir *Billy, Me & You* (2011) is about her process of bereavement following the death of her child. Nicola directs LDComics (est. 2009 as Laydeez do Comics), the international women-led comics forum open to all. Her AHRC-funded doctoral research informed her co-editing of *The Inking Woman* (2018), an illustrated history of women's cartooning in Britain for a general

reader. This is complemented by her publication *UK Feminist Cartoons and Comics: A Critical Survey* (2020). www.streetenillustration.com, @NicolaStreeten.

A. K. Summers is the author and artist of the graphic memoir *Pregnant Butch*, which was nominated for a 2015 Lambda Literary Award and included in *Best American Comics 2015* as a notable comic. She lives with her son in Providence, Rhode Island. www.aksummers.com.

Kimiko Tobimatsu is a lawyer born and raised in Toronto. She loves to play squash, search out delicious food, and attempt to be handy around the house. www.kimikodoescancer.com.

Carol Tyler is an award-winning American comics artist/writer known for her autobiographical stories. Her work has appeared in many publications and anthologies, such as the *Wimmens Comix, Twisted Sisters, LA Weekly*, and *Best American Comics*. Solo books include *The Job Thing* (1993), *Late Bloomer* (2005), the much-honored *Soldier's Heart: The Campaign to Understand My WWII Veteran Father* (2015), and *Fab4 Mania* (2018). Current book in progress: *The Ephemerata: Shaping the Exquisite Nature of My Grief*.

Shelley Wall is a medical illustrator and assistant professor in the biomedical communications graduate program at the University of Toronto, where she teaches courses in graphic medicine and in pathological, neuroanatomical, and bioscientific illustration. www.shelleywall.layfigures.com.

Dana Walrath, a writer, artist, and anthropologist, likes to cross borders and disciplines with her work. She spent 2012–13 as a Fulbright Scholar in Armenia completing *Like Water on Stone*, her award-winning verse novel about the Armenian genocide. Her graphic memoir, *Aliceheimer's*—about life with her mother, Alice, and dementia—was featured in the *New York Times*, the *Los Angeles Review of Books*, and on National Public Radio. Passionate about the power of art for social change, her installation *View from the High Ground* uses interactive artists' books to counter dehumanization and genocide. Illustrated essays and commentary have appeared in *The Lancet*, *Irish Times*, *Slate*, *Somatosphere*, *Foreign Policy*, and on public radio. She has spoken extensively about the healing power of stories throughout North America and Eurasia, including two TEDx talks. A Senior Atlantic Fellow for Equity in Brain Health at Trinity College Dublin | University of California San Francisco, she is currently working on a second *Aliceheimer's* book that will blend personal memoir with anthropological discourse on the end of life, stigma, gender, labor flows, and dementia across the globe.

editor

MK Czerwiec is a nurse, cartoonist, educator, and co-founder of the field of Graphic Medicine. She is the creator of *Taking Turns: Stories from HIV/AIDS Care Unit 371* (2017) and a co-author of *Graphic Medicine Manifesto* (2014). MK is also the comics editor for the journal *Literature & Medicine*. She regularly teaches graphic medicine at Northwestern University's Feinberg Medical School and the University of Chicago. MK has served as a Senior Fellow of the George Washington School of Nursing Center for Health Policy and Media Engagement as well as a Will Eisner Fellow in Applied Cartooning at the Center for Cartoon Studies in White River Junction, Vermont. You can see more of her work at her website, www.comic nurse.com.

Cataloging-in-Publication Data on file with the Library of Congress

The contributors to *Menopause: A Comic Treatment* retain copyright to their works in the volume, which appear here by permission. Teva Harrison's "The Big Change" is reproduced here with permission from House of Anansi. Further reproduction is prohibited.

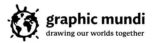

Graphic Mundi is an imprint of The Pennsylvania State University Press.

The Pennsylvania State University Press is a member of the Association of University Presses.

It is the policy of The Pennsylvania State University Press to use acid-free paper. Publications on uncoated stock satisfy the minimum requirements of American National Standard for Information Sciences—Permanence of Paper for Printed Library Material, ANSI z39.48–1992.